UNHOOKED

Inspiring Stories About Rebounds, Relapses and Successful Recoveries

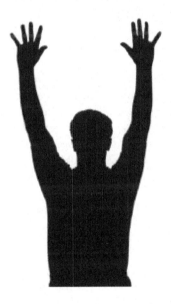

Compiled by Kathy Cournan Sarro

Publisher: Your Shift Matters Publishing, a Division of Dana Zarcone International, LLC
http://www.yourshiftmatters.com/

Book Cover and Formatting by Let's Get Booked
www.letsgetbooked.com

ISBN: 978-1-7378234-2-1

TABLE OF CONTENTS

INTRODUCTION

Drug addiction, drug overdoses, and drug-related deaths have become a pandemic across the globe. Every year, the numbers and the tears shed increases, and there is no end in sight. The number of drug-related deaths has increased at staggering rates. Many countries have tried different programs and strategies to change this trend. However, nothing has worked, and it continues to get worse.

America is at the forefront of this severe crippling epidemic. In 2021, there were over 100,000 reported deaths caused by drug overdoses. This number is staggering! That's almost twice as many people that died in the Vietnam War! Entire generations have been wiped out over this. Everyone seems to have been affected by drug addiction. It may be a neighbor, family member, co-worker, or friend. This epidemic does not discriminate. You can be rich, poor, black, white, Asian, male, female, Christian, Muslim, famous or unknown. There are no boundaries as to who may be affected… who may have the "monkey" on their back that comes with addiction.

Drug addiction comes with a hefty price for the addict, their families, and their friends. Not to mention the stranglehold it has on the economy. Active addiction changes a beautiful person into someone unrecognizable. When people are in active addiction, their thinking is so deranged. They don't think they are doing well, looking well, or functioning well. The truth is ugly. People that are in active addiction will do anything to get their drugs. They often hurt those that are closest to them just to get their next

1

fix. Genuinely good people do horrible things. Fortunately, once someone finds sobriety, they are able to become the good person they once were. In fact, many loved ones say, "It's nice to have my daughter/son/sister back."

So, what can be done to turn this epidemic around? There are treatments such as Methadone, Suboxone, Vivitrol, and Subutex. There are Alcoholics Anonymous and Narcotics Anonymous (AA/NA) meetings, church groups, Jesus Christ, and Buddha. The resources are out there. That said, when it comes to combating drug addiction, it takes a village.

Sober living communities are great because they provide doctors, therapy, support groups, social activities, work, and transportation. These types of facilities offer so much support that the success rate is much greater than trying to do it alone. It is important for anyone who struggles with addiction to tap into a strong support system so they can take the necessary steps to recover successfully. When support is scarce, recovery is much more difficult. Unfortunately, many people don't have support, and without support, problems are bound to get worse before they get better. As I said, it takes a village. A village that offers support, resources and services focused and committed to helping people do well, live well, and be well.

The purpose of this book is to enlighten people. To help people understand addiction from the addict's perspective so that they can become more compassionate and understanding. Addiction is an uncontrollable, horrible disease. Many people don't understand why or how people become addicts. They mistakenly believe that people who become addicted to drugs or alcohol lack strength, willpower, or moral principles. They think that if an addict wanted to stop using, they could simply choose to stop. Nothing could be further from the truth.

Drug addiction is a complex disease, and recovery usually takes something much more than the right mindset, good intentions, or split decision. Drugs change the brain and makes recovery difficult. Fortunately, there are so many programs and treatments available that people who want to recover from drug addiction can do so successfully and go on to live productive, happy lives.

Personally, I have an adult child with severe mental retardation. There seem to be many parallels, which is why I can relate to their struggles on such a deep level. There are a lot of negative opinions and judgements about addicts and the path they choose to get clean. It shouldn't matter what path they choose. They may choose to go to church meetings, participate in a Methadone or Suboxone program, check into an inpatient treatment facility… it doesn't matter. What matters most is that they find the strength and courage to deal with their addiction and that they do… get clean! The path someone chooses doesn't matter as long as it works.

I am not saying that everyone who sets out to recover from addiction is successful. There is no "cookie cutter" solution and there certainly isn't a magic wand or an easy button either. There are people out there who, deep down, do not want to change so recovery will be virtually impossible. If someone does not want sobriety, it's never going to happen. Period.

All I am asking is that we keep an open mind. That we open our hearts, and we support the people that are willing to change.

Support those that are willing to do the work… regardless of the recovery path they choose.

I can tell you many stories of people who hide their recovery because their family members don't want them in a program. They know they have to get into a recovery program because it's the only way they can stop using, become sober and responsible. Yet they can't talk to people about it because of the criticism and judgements that have to endure. Getting sober is hard enough without being judged, put down, and criticized. I've seen people leave treatment because of this and a few months later they are at the funeral home.

I've compiled this book of stories written by brave, courageous people from all walks of life that are willing to share their battles with addiction. Some of these people have passed. Some continue to struggle. Many have recovered and continue to do well.

This book is intended to honor the people who have suffered with addiction as well as the people out there who are supporting them on their journey. To all the people who wrote their stories, God bless you. It is my hope that by sharing these stories, we can inspire people… maybe even save a few.

Whatever people are going through, we should always be kind and supportive. Is life fair? No, it's not. But it could always be worse. Always be grateful. My son is twenty-eight years old, and he has taught me to be grateful. I agree it can be difficult at times, but we should try to be grateful, and appreciate the kindness of others, as much as possible. One person can make a difference. Let it be you.

Never underestimate the power of one kind word, a friendly smile, or a kind gesture. They can make a huge difference in someone's life. These simple things can have a huge impact... especially for someone who is suffering.

My challenge to you is to be that person that makes a difference. Be that someone who will take anything negative and turn it into something positive. Be supportive of people you know that may be suffering from addiction. Open your mind, open your hearts... smile, you are beautiful.

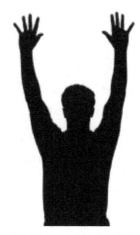

CHAPTER ONE

Now I Lay Me Down to Sleep

By John

"I understood myself only after I destroyed myself. And only in the process of fixing myself, did I know who I really was."

– Unknown

Hello, my name is John, and I am a recovering addict.

I have been gifted with an opportunity to share my journey of addiction and recovery with you. This is a chance for me to reach people in extraordinary pain and show that it's possible to transform your life. I aim to touch as many people's hearts and souls as possible. If you are in pain and can't see a way out of the misery and turmoil, please open your mind to what I have to share with you. The dark, hopeless abyss you're helplessly trapped in is no way to live. If you're contemplating change yet unsure how to do it, or if it's even possible, please read on as I prove to you that it is.

I'm originally from Pittsburgh, Pa, but I have lived in many places over my thirty-four years. I've been in a very long battle with addiction from thirteen to thirty-four. I felt like a prisoner of war most of my life. I could never understand why I had been dealt the hand in a game I had no business playing. I was now a player in the game of life without a strategy or knowing how to play. But, as with most things in life, I learned fast and would become one hell of a card player.

My story begins with horrific, non-suppressed childhood memories that haunt me daily. Over years and years of trauma, rage, and addiction, I was conditioned to only see the negative in life. Pessimism is always seeing things as half empty, never half full. This has been my attitude toward most things in life. It should be easy to see why, yet it's not impossible to change.

My earliest memories are very descriptive and may trigger some people. It's not my intention to offend anyone or convince you I am a victim, although I believed I was for many years and even learned to use it to my advantage. During my childhood, I was exposed to a lot of drug use and drug deals. I also recall the horrible words that were said to my mother and me. Some of the words would be played back in my mind, forever stuck on repeat. I was the victim of physical, mental, and sexual abuse. Men usually don't admit the latter, especially when it was done to them by a woman. I was physically beaten almost every day by an extensive list of my mother's men and by her. I was always in the wrong place at the wrong time. I saw a lot of things that I should never have seen. Acts I have only begun to describe.

The first prayer I ever said, besides "now I lay me down to sleep," went something like, "God, please end my life. I do not understand why you allow me to go through this. If you do not take me in my sleep tonight, I'll know you're not real, and your power is not real... just like Santa and those little elves aren't real." It was the holiday season. I was told to stop being an idiot and grow up. I was also told Santa and his elves were all fake and never to believe in such nonsense. This was Christmas Eve, 1993, during one of the biggest blizzards on record. I had been praying, consciously crying out for help long before a substance entered my body.

I wanted to catch Santa eating the cookie I left out for him by the tree. So I tried to sneak past the people doing little white lines off the kitchen counter and smoking these long glass cigarettes. Unfortunately, I got caught on my way back up the stairs to my bedroom. I remember those words being drilled into me as I was hit over my head and body. The weapon of choice was a 24-inch wooden paddle made from a 2x4 with holes drilled into it. I don't know if the holes were in it to increase the speed of the swing or if it was for the sound effect I can still hear to this very day. This was a recurring theme throughout my childhood. However, sometimes the weapons varied, including pots and pans, extension cords, and belts.

One night, I was told to hide. "Hurry, hurry, don't make a sound or let anyone know you're here. Please, Johnny, no matter what happens, don't come out until I come and get you." So, I ran for my favorite hiding place. It was a small access panel for plumbing in the back of my mother's bedroom closet. I remember hearing "he's not here." and "I don't have the money to pay you." The next thing I heard were screams of terror coming from my mother as she was beaten and dragged into the bedroom.

I crawled out just enough to look through the shutter doors. Two men were holding her down, laughing as they ravaged her. The third assailant raped her. I wanted to save her, but I was afraid of what they would do to me. I couldn't bring myself to break the promise I made to my mother about staying hidden. Another man used my mother for a place to stay, sex, drugs, and all our money. Like so many before, he had left all the wreckage behind for my mother to clean up. We decided to move, and my grandfather got us a place in east Pittsburgh called Braddock.

I made no effort to make friends usually. I was only eight years old and knew we would not stay there long. We rarely did. My father was never really involved in my life much back then. He had a falling out with my mother, and they divorced when I was very young. I found out much later in life that he tried to get custody of me, and it did not pan out well. I often wonder if that would have made a difference. He remarried a mutual friend of theirs. My mother would never forgive him for that. She went out of her way to make me believe my father was a liar, cheater, and evil. I knew better.

My father was introduced to recovery after a long hard run of selling and using cocaine. In my opinion, this is what brought my mother and father together. I visited with my father before 1993 and after 1997. He was introduced to a program that saved his life and sanity. I was not sure why he was not involved in my life much. Did he not want me, either? Later I found out that he had to stay away from my mother to stay clean and sober. They were toxic to each other, and my mother would use me against him for years.

As a result of my father's absence, I had severe abandonment issues. I couldn't understand why my father didn't want anything to do with me. Why was my mother always too busy to spend any time with me? I watched other families with envy and confusion. Was I such a bad kid? Was I ugly? Why was I not wanted? These questions became the basis for a belief system I later referred to as 'toxic shame.'

I went through my childhood feeling confused, less than, and worthless. These negative beliefs were instilled in me from such a young age. Deep down, I thought I was an idiot, useless, stupid, and would never amount to anything. I was often told, "Even your dad doesn't want you." I truly believed them with all my heart. As a result, I became very resentful at a very early age.

During my short stay in Braddock, I watched my mother sell herself for drugs. I remember being left at a park while she went off with a few people to make money. I still remember how confused I was seeing other children with loving parents. What made these children so much better than me?

I was physically, mentally, and emotionally abused for over twenty years. This had a significant impact on my decision-making abilities. As a result, my main focus was filling the void and getting attention and acceptance from others throughout my life.

Christmas seems to be the season for trauma and degradation, so I lack holiday cheer at that time of the year. My next vivid memory was on another Christmas Eve. I was given a large tin can with three different flavors of popcorn. It was something I was going to save and share with my mother when she found time to watch a movie with me. I waited for what felt like forever, but it was probably just a few days.

Before we could find time to watch our movie together, a fight ensued. My mother was thrown headfirst into our large tin popcorn can and was bleeding out on the living room floor. Once again, she lay before me in a drunken pool of blood and tears. When she looked up at me, I could see the pain, fear, and agony in her eyes. I had enough. I couldn't sit on the sidelines anymore. For the first time, I lost all sense of fear. It no longer immobilized me. I attacked the man with a baseball bat, a gift he gave me.

I was a big kid and a good athlete, so I smashed him hard and as many times as I could before exhaustion set in, and I knew I got my point across. Finally, the police showed up, and he was hauled away in an ambulance. I finally felt like I had a purpose. I want to do this from now on… hurt people who picked on the less fortunate. I would become the valiant white knight, the protector of my mother and my loving baby sister, the daughter of that evil man. My desire to protect people would become my focus for years to come. As you'll later learn, it became my justification for things I did that I still regret today.

I now know my mother wasn't the only one trapped in a vicious cycle of insanity. Her addiction to drugs, alcohol, and evil men was never-ending. Eventually, our lives would become intertwined. I began to embrace my own self-hatred, anger, and rage. I adopted a toxic belief system that would take years to unravel. But, like my mother, I had no idea I had begun to spiral downhill. I was oblivious to everything going on in my tiny little world.

As years passed, many other destructive cycles would get added to my typhoon of life. Eventually, I will begin to understand what was happening to us. If only I knew then what I know now. Does everything happen the way it's supposed to? Or is it my option to view it how I wish?

I admit that I focused more on my external motivators than my internal ones. How I thought people perceived me would be a building block for how I would make choices in my life. Being raised the way I was, I was ashamed, embarrassed, belittled, and ridiculed for as long as I can remember. As a result, I got into role-playing and people-pleasing. I always had a variety of masks to choose from. I like to think of the masks as my survival instincts taking over, similar to poker when you have to bluff. I didn't want people to be able to read me or really see me.

I didn't want them to see the deeper feelings or root emotions I was experiencing. After many years of practice, I had become successfully numb. I had become entranced in a state of anhedonia.

This cycle continues throughout my life and shows up in more areas than just where I choose to call home. I lose interest in things quickly, including jobs, women, cars, new cities, and my hobbies. I feel at times like I just need more excitement. Life gets bland and monotonous when you're always doing the same thing. I was bored and addicted to chaos. The constant need for excitement. Of course, this got me into a boatload of trouble.

Eventually, we moved from Braddock to the inner city of Pittsburgh, a small section in Lawrenceville's 9th ward. Starting in a new school, I could set a standard. I needed to let people know that I meant business and wouldn't take crap from anyone! After all, they had no clue that I just beat a man over with a baseball bat!

I made a few friends very quickly. I was shown parts of town I had no business being in. We would skip school, swim in the river, and vandalize parks and bridges. I was acting out and becoming comfortable with things I had never done before. My morals and values were beginning to change. I was starting to lose myself to others. I loved the adrenaline rush and thrill of doing something wrong. What if we get caught running away from the scene of the crime? I would soon get the attention I had always wanted, just from the wrong people.

It was Halloween, and my mom wanted to take me trick or treating. We had a big English springer who would join us. I was so impatient that night because it took forever to get ready to go. My mom needed one more beer, a bathroom break, and one more beer. I remember thinking all the candy would be gone by the time we left the house. So why couldn't I just go with my friends? After all, I am a big boy now.

We finally left, walked one block, and the next thing I knew, she was flailing on the ground. Our dog had pulled her down, trying to get to someone she recognized. My mother smashed her face on the curb. At this point in my life, I was losing my patience. My desire to protect her had all but vanished. I had become enraged

13

and embarrassed that she had found a way to do this to me yet again. Long story short, that was the end of my Halloween experience that year.

I had become so resentful and angry because I was dealt some pretty crappy hands throughout my life. I couldn't understand why my mother wouldn't stop drinking and drugging. Her struggles were a mystery to me until I experienced this myself. So many people judged me and made fun of me... 'the drunk's son'. Kids would say very mean things that made me feel completely inferior. They would say, "That is the crackhead's boy! Look at his shoes and clothes. Mommy must have smoked and drank away all of the money."

This made me beyond angry! People needed to learn who I really was and what I could do to them. Eventually, I was kicked out of three schools and arrested for vandalizing houses and cars. After that, I was always in the doghouse. Then, on one particular day, I was grounded and sent to my room, and they told me to watch my sister.

They put her in my room, closed the door, and then placed a padlock on my door. We were prisoners in our own home. Apparently, my mother and her new boyfriend thought going to Graceland, Tennessee, was a good idea. I had no idea when or if they were coming home. I tried everything I could to bust down the door. Not an easy feat when you're dealing with thick oak doors and padlocks. My sister and I were starving. We used a trash can as a toilet, and I had no idea what to do next. The only thing I could do was scold God yet again. I called Him all kinds of names and said things I won't repeat here. Let's just say my vocabulary had become quite extensive.

I had worn myself out. I was physically and mentally exhausted. At one point, I finally fell asleep. My little sister had been in tears for days, asking where our mother was. "Is she coming back, Johnny? What do we do? I'm so hungry?" She decided to climb out our second-story window while I was sleeping. I am so grateful she didn't fall to her death that day. The screaming woke me up. What was happening? Had my mother returned, or was it one of my nightmares again? I didn't know. I couldn't tell what was real anymore.

I was overwhelmed with fear and panic as I saw her little fingers holding on to the windowsill. Two old ladies were screaming and pounding on our door. They had no idea we had been locked in that room for days with nobody to care for us.

The police and fire trucks came to our rescue, and we were sent to my grandparents' house. My grandparents were alcoholics and fought a lot, but it was not nearly as bad as at my mom's house.

While living with my grandparents, I had a lot more freedom. I played the victim to manipulate people into getting my way. I was twelve years old, and it was the summer of 1998. I was introduced to marijuana and started stealing booze from my grandparents. The neighborhood kids loved me because I had an unlimited supply of vodka. I felt like people respected me and looked up to me. I finally found a solution for the pain, low self-esteem, anxiety, fear, resentment, and anger. Drugs and alcohol made me feel like I was on top of the world. I finally had friends who looked at me like I was somebody. Finally, I arrived! No one called me 'the crackhead's son.' People didn't speak to me that way because of what they witnessed me do when I was enraged.

I would now become an advanced-level card player at the ripe old age of thirteen! I learned how to fill my need for adrenaline and chaos. I found out a great deal of money could be made stealing cars. The thrill of stealing was enticing. But stealing fast cars when I wasn't old enough to drive appealed to me even more. I found ways to fuel my desires by any means necessary. Stealing, using, selling, fighting, running away for days on end, causing mischief... all of it had become my new reality.

I was now using my family's connections to build my reputation. Who would suspect a thirteen-year-old kid of being a drug dealer? I was always around the older crowd at the park, the river, drinking and using. I was well known for having money, connections, and products most people couldn't get. I had a new set of friends, business associates, and views on the world around me. My mother is the first person I ever did cocaine with. One evening, she told me, "Johnny, if you ever want to try any drugs or drink, I prefer you do it here, so I know you're safe." I couldn't wait to take her up on her offer.

Mother and her friends could no longer control me. I was in charge and made the rules now. I was a part of the family and part of the crowd. I continued to make reckless decisions. I adopted the idea that I was a man now and free to make my own choices and rules. I loved the power and control I had over people... especially those who had power and control over me for so long. I had people who needed me, yes me, for the first time ever! My uncle, family and friends depended on me to get them what they needed. I was important to them now and had a new sense of purpose in life. The dealer dealt a new game of cards, and I needed to learn how to play fast!

As you're reading my story, you may be able to relate to some of this. I'm not trying to glorify my drug use or my life. Instead, I want you to understand the lessons I learned the hard way in hopes that they will help you understand the journey of an addict.

I was living in a world full of delusions of grandeur. I only saw the world through one set of lenses. I firmly believed that this metaphoric card game of life was the only life I would ever know. I was determined to become the best and most fierce person I could become. So I discovered new ways to play the game.

Eventually, I was thrown out of school, on the news, and on the run from law enforcement. I was technically homeless. I always had a place to stay, yet I couldn't go home because the law was looking for me. I had pending charges and was on the run since my first juvenile placement at the Academy. I escaped because I refused to be controlled or told what to do. Who did these people think they were, telling me how to live my life?!

I assaulted someone and decided that my only option was to run. I couldn't let them catch me. I didn't want to change, and I didn't want a 'better life.' How bland and boring that all seemed! I needed the adrenaline rush.

My mother wanted me to turn myself in, and, after a very long summer, I realized a few things:

1. It was terrible having to run from the police all the time.

2.   I couldn't go back to school, get an education, or a driver's license.

3.   I wanted to go to college just to party, and I never planned on getting a career or decent job.

People in my world just made it through life hustling and stealing. Unfortunately, these were things I was addicted to and pretty good at.

Somehow my mother talked me into turning myself in. Who was I kidding? I turned myself in because I thought I would get less time. I was in a maximum-security juvenile detention center for six months. Then, on my fourteenth birthday, I was transferred to an all-boys non-profit residential treatment facility. Wow, was I a nuisance and menace to society! They had no idea what was in store for them.

I remember walking in like a tough guy, so everyone knew I was not to be toyed with. But the truth is I was really terrified. I didn't want people to take something I had, and I feared I wouldn't get my way. Things wouldn't happen the way I wanted them to. I had very little control and hated that I wasn't in charge. So I tried to run the show and control the game.

That facility probably saved my life even though I hated most of it. It would be four years to the day before I would get to leave. I guess that's what I deserved for stealing the sheriff's car and making the news during a huge school fight.

During the first year, I was in their lockdown facility. I had chased a parent with a chair and flipped out because I didn't get my way. Sorry, Mr. Aaron, I had no idea how to deal with my emotions back then. Everything came out as rage and hatred. But really, I was only mad at myself and the big guy upstairs. God had yet again betrayed me and put me into this hell hole.

It had always been easy to point fingers and blame others for my problems; after all, I had nothing to do with it. Finally, after being there for almost a year, I was told to get out to the main campus. I would have to agree to do one hundred and eighty hours of community service. I told them to go to hell, of course. I had no intention of working ever… let alone for free. These people were out of their minds! I told them, "You can't keep me here forever! You'll have to let me go one day." This was my attitude toward most things in life, defiant to the end.

A month later, this woman came in to speak with me. I was very unsure of her. She was not easy to read, and I was confused about why she asked to talk to me. I assumed she was a doctor or psychiatrist, but I had never seen one dress like she did. I noticed she was in dirty jeans and cowboy boots. Her top was red and black flannel, and she seemed rugged. I felt I could trust this woman for some reason, so I agreed to chat. I was comfortable around her. She seemed like 'my kind of people.'

She asked me what I liked to do. This stumped me. I had so many questions for her but didn't want to answer any of her questions. Finally, we agreed that if I answered one question of hers, she would answer two of mine. How could I refuse? The odds were in my favor!

I shrugged my shoulders and asked her who she was. She reminded me that I had to answer one of her questions for two questions answered in return. A shrug of the shoulders would not suffice. Damn, she was good! I thought, "No getting over on her!" I told her I liked swimming in the river and partying with my friends. She didn't respond or make a face at me like most people do when I have a slick answer. Instead, Mrs. Debbie, this rugged woman, just said, "I used to love doing that also."

Now she had me confused. Was I about to be rescued by a woman who liked partying and swimming?! We talked for an hour or two, and I eventually opened up to her... even I was surprised. She never judged me or made me feel 'less than'.

She told me if I agreed to do my community service with her, she would help me get outside, and I would get to work with animals. She had a horse barn on campus with 27 horses and needed my help with them. This was a hard decision for me. Someone needing my help was questionable, to say the least. What did she really want?

By this time, I had learned that people always had ulterior motives, especially me. I did not want to shovel horse dung! These horses were big dirty animals! Were they dangerous? This kind of appealed to me, actually. It wasn't a car, but I loved being outdoors, and they were fast, too! I have always enjoyed animals! These animals deserved respect. They didn't yell at me or talk back; they just loved unconditionally.

I agreed to help her despite my reservations about all the work I would have to do. But, she promised to show me how to ride, and I always wanted to learn how to ride a horse!

Even though I was 'working' now, I still managed to find trouble. My mother was able to visit a few times, showing up drunk on several occasions. She would bring me contraband that I could sell on campus. I was so addicted to the lifestyle and the adrenaline that came with it that I couldn't stop.

We weren't allowed to smoke or chew tobacco products... so I started selling them. Eventually, I started selling porn magazines, drugs, lighters, and other paraphernalia. I even manipulated a staff member into bringing me things I could sell or use. I got really good at smuggling the contraband onto campus. I had my mother put it in a giant tree stump down behind the horse pastures. Later, I'd take a walk or trail ride to get it and bring it back to campus. Riding was quite beneficial! We weren't allowed to have money, yet somehow, I left with over five thousand dollars in my pocket two years later.

I hid the cash and contraband in the same area until my eighteenth birthday when I could go back and get it and not be stopped. At eighteen, I wouldn't be under anyone's control anymore. I would be a man.

I started developing a conscience. I felt empathy and compassion when I was working with these magnificent creatures. Mrs. Debbie and I developed a bond I had never experienced before. She was like a mother to me. I longed for the love I never had growing up and found it! I felt terrible that I was doing such bad things. I was betraying her trust and love for me when she was doing so much to help me. I felt guilt and shame for my actions for the first time ever. I did not want to feel that way anymore. Who would? It sucks!

I needed to escape from reality. I had a few friends that were in placement with me. They were confidants of mine and helped me in my pursuit to make money. We discussed a plan to escape. We would steal the night guard's car and leave him tied up so he couldn't tell anybody. I've never told anyone until now.

A couple of nights before our escape, I couldn't sleep. I had an inner voice saying, "This is a bad idea. You only have a few months to go until you're eighteen." For some reason, I couldn't bring myself to run. I would have to leave Mrs. Debbie and the horses behind. What would she think of me? Would it hurt her? I no longer wanted to cause pain or harm anyone, and my time there was almost up.

This was the first time I listened to that little voice inside me. It was my own Jiminy Cricket that saved my life that night. Unfortunately, the other boys murdered that guard that night. They beat him with socks filled with batteries and soap. They were later caught and arrested.

I laid in bed many nights, romanticizing my drug use and dreaming up ways to make money. I couldn't wait to get out and start consuming and selling drugs again. Finally, I could make some real money, not just petty cash. I kept thinking about how the drugs will take away all the pain. Being under the influence was the only time I was free from my feelings and emotions. After all these years, I was still consumed by my urges and desires. I was thoroughly obsessed with using and not feeling. I never learned how to deal with my emotions. I usually did it via violent outbursts and didn't see myself changing.

I made up my mind that my life was never going to change. That it was going to be the way it always was. I didn't see a way out or have any desire to change. I was blind in so many areas. I didn't know that I was digging a hole that would be nearly impossible to climb out of. So I got back into the game, intending to win the jackpot.

When I got home to Pittsburgh, everyone welcomed me with open arms. My welcome home gift was an ankle bracelet, a pound of weed, and a few ounces of cocaine. Except for the ankle monitor, I thought it was the greatest gift ever! I would unplug my box and go out all night. I never passed one urine test and had thousands of reasons to get in trouble. Yet, somehow, I was able to get off of house arrest.

I discovered if the phone was off the hook and rang busy, they couldn't trace my whereabouts. So, I would go out and party all night long and have call forwarding on my cell phone if they ever called. I was right back in the middle of the chaos I longed for. The game didn't really change, but the players sure had. It took me a while to see through people's bluffs and fronts and get to know who I was now playing with.

My grandmother ended up in a nursing home with cirrhosis of the liver and was paralyzed on her left side. So, I inherited the house, and my grandparents moved to another place on the river. I was deep into being an addict and selling drugs. At one point, I was stabbed in the back on my front porch, the first of many stabbings.

I experienced my first overdose of heroin and started smoking crack cocaine. My house became a one-stop-shop and was always full of people. I had people from different walks of life with one common denominator, drugs.

I was incarcerated just six months after being released from juvenile. I had been in jail about twenty-two times by the time I was twenty-one. Eventually, I was doing more of my product than

23

I was selling. Rule number one: don't get high on your own supply! Apparently, I missed that memo.

My father received a call from police in October of 2008 stating that I was in the back of their car for stealing pharmaceuticals. He pleaded with the officers to release me. Thankfully, the place I had robbed decided not to press charges. I assumed it was due to my reputation and fears of retaliation.

As a person in recovery himself, my poor father had done so much for me. This man spent hundreds of thousands of dollars on bail bonds, lawyers, housing, and fines. He felt that if I stayed in Pittsburgh, I would die. So, he got me a place in Butler County, gave me a job at his business, and things went well for a brief time. I was no longer doing hard drugs, but I was still smoking pot and drinking. I would now try to control my use and limit substances for the first time ever.

Over the years, I've learned my problems come from within, not in the world that I live in. Soon, a woman was hired that liked to drink. I went to a party with her and stayed at her place that night. We had a great time. One of my best memories, to be honest. However, neither one of us showed up to work the next day.

My father was banging on my door to no avail. Finally, he put two and two together and showed up at her house in an uproar. Mind you, my father is not an easy man to upset. This time, he was so upset that he got a restraining order. I wasn't allowed on company property anymore. That said, my father and I have a decent relationship today. He is a great man and has continued to inspire me and lead by example despite all I've done over the years. I love you, dad. Thank you for never giving up on me!

The last day I worked for my father was May 10th, 2009, Mother's Day. I had moved my mother into the house my grandfather left me. Eventually, she and her boyfriend filed a restraining order against me because I assaulted him several times. These monsters taught me more than I realized. A seed was planted in me, which eventually took root. I deserved to lose my place, and I lost a lot of respect for myself and my mother. I couldn't understand why she continued to do this to herself and allowed these monsters to be in her life.

When I was twenty-two, I decided to see my mother again. I got her a card and flowers. I wanted to let her know I was doing better and hoped she was. But, when I got there, the house gave me the chills. I could barely breathe as I approached the door. I shook uncontrollably like Bruce Banner about to transform into the incredible hulk.

I had to go through the kitchen window to get into the house. My mother was beaten and battered head to toe. Her head was as swollen as a basketball, and her leg was in a cast. What was once my grandparents' beautiful home was now littered with empty pill bottles, beer, and vodka bottles. The house reeked of alcohol and smoke, like a dive bar in the middle of nowhere. I had flashbacks of my suppressed childhood experiences at that moment. I saw nothing but red and demanded she tells me who had done this to her. She wouldn't tell me, so I called her a few choice names and stormed out of the house... never to return again.

I was on a mission to find out who had done this. Feeling this level of pain and agony was no longer an option anymore. I was in pain like never before and was just a block or two away from what I knew would take it all away. Off I went. To this day, I have no idea how I got back home, but I showed up for work the next day. Before lunch, I got pulled into the office by my father and uncle. I could tell something was wrong. They told me they got a call from the county coroner… my mother was gone. Her cause of death was 'unknown.'

I don't remember feeling anything, really. I just remember my dad chasing after me, telling me not to leave. We both knew what would happen, and there was no way to stop what was being unleashed inside me.

Within an hour or two, I had a gun and loads of drugs. I wanted to know who killed my mother and find him. It had to be a man. It always was. I emptied my bank account and told my dad to keep the place and everything in it. I remember the look he gave me as he watched me leave. He didn't know if he would ever see me again.

I had no intention of surviving or letting my mother's killer survive. I got the information I needed and went on the hunt. The man I was looking for is no longer with us today. He took his own life because of what he had done to my mother. He couldn't live with himself. As I sat there looking at his corpse, anger and resentment filled my heart. I thought about dismembering and mutilating his corpse.

Regardless of where I was, I had one purpose… to get drugs and make money by any means necessary. I was on probation in three counties and didn't care if they ever saw me again. Off to the races would be putting it lightly. I wanted to die and did everything in my power to make it happen, except squeeze the trigger myself. I couldn't come to terms with reality. My worst childhood fears had taken hold of me. My mother was gone and never coming back.

I blamed myself for not being there for her. I was the white knight, the brave protector, the failure. Where was I, and what had I done? I couldn't see how I had let this happen. In the end, revenge was stolen from me. Anger couldn't touch the pure hatred I had for myself. I despised God for what He had done. But, even more so, I hated myself for not staying with her and saving her. I wanted to die every waking moment, and the only thing that helped was the next fix or the adrenaline rush when I took chances with my life.

I consumed more drugs in one day than most people do in weeks. I had to do more and more to dull the pain. I was fearless in my attempts to obtain more, no matter the cost. I sold my services to bookies, women, and dealers larger than myself. The drugs were my only escape from reality... my only way to survive.

I was a monster back then. I do not allow it to control me, though. I made selfish choices and caused so much harm to others. What hurts most is the innocent people I've hurt along the way. They probably have post-traumatic stress disorder (PTSD) because of me. In fact, I suffer from a very complex form of PTSD and would not wish it on my worst enemy.

In November 2014, my dad talked me into returning to Pennsylvania. But unfortunately, I was not equipped to deal with my demons and what was yet to come.

I got a job with my dad's friend from church. I got an apartment and other things I didn't deserve. This was great, but then I experienced the worst detox in my entire life. I lay in my bed kicking, shaking, sweating, and spasming uncontrollably. The hallucinations were real, and the trauma trapped inside for years spewed out of me. My neighbors called the police because I was screaming in my sleep... and again when I was awake. I thought people were coming for me, and they knew where I was. I was still trying to save my mother, but it was impossible. She would yell at me in my dreams, "Why didn't you save me? You're a terrible son, an abomination! I should never have had you!"

After just a month at work, I couldn't take it anymore. One day, my boss handed me my paycheck, and I said, "Thank you for everything, but I quit! Don't worry, I'll be fine. Go back home and tell my dad I'm leaving, and please don't try to stop me."

I have always been great at quitting. I would quit if I didn't want to work hard on something. I quit smoking a thousand times and quit drugs a thousand more. The hardest part is sticking to it. This separates the men from the boys, as they say.

I didn't have a bank account or any identification, and I needed a way to cash my last check. So, I went to a friend's pizza shop, where I used to work. He knew he could trust me. The man who owned this fine establishment happened to be one of the bookies I worked for.

He would move a lot of stolen goods for me over the years and had deep pockets. Many of my acquaintances did too, which is why my addiction continued for many years. I could always find a way to get more. I always had a solution. I had become one hell of a problem solver. My motivation was always geared towards getting high and getting whatever I wanted. Drugs and alcohol were my 'go-to solution.' As silly as it may sound, the drugs really saved my life. My problems weren't the drugs and alcohol. That's how I coped. My problems were because of the relationship I had with myself.

I experienced many blackouts over the years, and I discovered not all of them directly resulted from using drugs. Triggered traumatic events caused me to blackout too. As a result, I lost days, weeks, and even months.

I'd wake up to a few girls and lots of leftover drugs. I had no idea how I got back to my place. I had no idea what I had done or who the two women were lying in my bed. Someone was beating on my door, and I just sat there, appreciating the moment a little longer. I didn't want to come back to reality. Before I opened the door, I consumed a large quantity of whatever was lying around and opened the door. I guess I had been busy the night before. I had two high-stakes players with duffle bags full of goodies at my door. Apparently, the night before, we agreed to set up shop in our town.

By march of 2015, I had lost myself yet again. I robbed all the dealers and had seven girls working for me, who later saved my life. I was experiencing physical and spiritual death, but I didn't know it at the time. I had allowed these women to act like my mother and justified it by being their protector.

I had a blood infection from dirty needles. My hand was as big as a softball. I ended up going septic, and my organs shut down on me. One woman I was protecting called for help when I collapsed. I woke up in the hospital for the third time in four months. The first time, I was stabbed in the head. The second time was due to a blood infection. The third time, I had sepsis. This is when you have an infection, and your body turns on itself, resulting in severe organ damage and, usually, death.

I'm not quite sure why my life was spared so many times over the years. But, I know today that my story will help save many lives and hopefully, it will be an inspiration for people to change.

When I woke up in the hospital, I was hooked up to all sorts of machines and breathing tubes. I had a pneumothorax, which is a collapsed lung. I was in so much pain despite the medications I was on. My tolerance for opioids was quite substantial. My liver was in terrible shape, having reinfected myself with hepatitis C... once again. My body was shutting down, and how it endured years of abuse is beyond me.

Doctors and nurses looked at me in a way that still haunts me today. I was stubborn and caught up in my addiction, self-pity, and self-hatred. I hated my life so much that I didn't fear death. This has been a constant theme in my life. When I don't want to deal with life or feel my emotions, my solution is to get numb.

I was only in the hospital for an hour before I started making some calls. I had people bringing me what I longed for and felt I couldn't survive without. I would shoot heroin into my antibiotic pic line. I smoked crack in the hospital room and bathroom. Eventually, a nurse found empty stamp bags on my bed, plus a used syringe. I obviously passed out before cleaning up after myself.

The hospital could have had me removed or arrested, but they didn't. They knew I needed help. They informed my father and uncle, and I couldn't have any more visitors except my immediate family. The family who would never bring me what I wanted the most. My girls weren't allowed to visit either, and I was outraged.

My father and his friend from church came to visit me. The moment they laid eyes on me, they began weeping. They had their Bibles and wanted to pray and read with me. If other people couldn't visit me, why could they? Why did they have a right to be here? I yelled at them and told them they needed to leave.

A few hours later, I panicked and decided it was time for me to go. I removed the IVs, tubes, and breathing apparatus and stumbled down the hall. The drugs were calling me. If I had to choose between getting my next fix, or my next breath of air, the choice was obvious... the fix. I managed to slip past security and hook up with my friends waiting for me at the emergency room entrance. Then, I was off to the races again.

My court dates were still pending, and probation and parole officers were looking for me. I had no intention of going back to jail or surviving long enough for them to catch me. So I skipped out on the bail and my hearings. I knew they would take me if I showed up, which would never happen.

I ended up robbing another drug dealer in the area and was going to break down what I could use and what I would sell. As soon as I got the scale and baggies out, I did a blast, then heard a bang. I didn't wait around to find out what it was. I could only assume it was either the police or a pissed-off dealer and his crew. It was the police. Somebody had informed them where I was.

I threw everything I could in my backpack, jumped out the window, shimmied up between the two houses, and scaled the walls to get to the roof. I jumped from one roof to another, then ducked behind a chimney. I had such a rush of adrenaline that it was a calling to my sick mind.

The police and swat team surrounded the whole block, and dogs circled on the ground below. As I watched them, I contemplated my escape, but part of me wanted to surrender. I just didn't want to run anymore. So, I sat there and smoked my product until the fire department arrived.

I was experiencing cocaine-induced paranoia, which made me do completely and utterly irrational, ridiculous things. I have never been right in the head, but I took insanity to a whole new level that morning.

After smoking most of the product a little while later, I diluted what was left in the puddles on the rooftop just before they convinced me there was no escape. So, I went down willingly.

I went through the worst withdrawal of my life and contemplated suicide many nights as I lay on my steel rack. My chase and rooftop standoff ended up on the news, in the paper, and on Facebook. Within my first two weeks in jail, I had accumulated five felonies: one burglary, possession of a firearm, and a slew of other charges. I knew I could not escape this one and would be going away for a long time.

I wanted to die. However, despite my thoughts of self-harm or suicide, I have not been one to act on them intentionally. I had been trying to kill myself most of my life, but it was never a conscious choice. That said, I was not trying to live either. Maybe I lacked conviction in my desire to die. Maybe there was something greater at work. Perhaps it goes back to when I said that prayer as a child. Who really knows.

I got sentenced to six to twelve years in prison. Once in jail and the toxins were out of my system, I had no choice but to face my demons. As many people do, I had the option to use drugs in jail, but without needles, why bother?

I was denied for the Selective Intervention Program (SIP) due to violence on my record and the nine warrants issued against me. I was wanted in four counties for a whole host of things. Apparently, I had been driving a stolen truck toward oncoming traffic and almost hit a police cruiser. I have no recollection of this event.

I was giving up on life and myself. I would never win or get ahead in life. This was my destiny, as I saw it. As previously stated, I could only see the world through one set of lenses. I was a programmed and conditioned pessimist. I was sitting in prison with no way out, carrying the guilt and shame I had felt for years. I was just as bad, if not worse, than the monsters I had encountered. I had to accept that fact. I almost convinced myself that this was what I deserved, but the determination to fight reared its ugly head again.

I got some of my self-confidence back shortly after my pity party. I would get out of this somehow because I am smart and won't let them win. I will find a way out, and so I did. I was determined to fight, and I stood resolute when that decision was made in my mind. Win, lose or draw, I would make my stand and let them know who they were dealing with.

I studied in the law library for weeks. I finally had a plan and some trump cards in my hand now. I set up an appeal and wrote a motion for another hearing stating I was misled and had an unfair trial. I also had a public defender, but I decided to represent myself and speak from the heart to this judge.

The judge granted my motion and hearing. I would soon have my sentence vacated... for the most part. I would get time served, paroled, sent back home, and, eventually, to a treatment facility.

I had weaseled my way out of all of that. I knew nobody was going to testify against me in court. I also knew that most of my victims were addicts, dealers, or dead. After all, I was not out there robbing upstanding citizens. So, I took a chance, and it paid off.

I was taking all the credit once again. I was the mastermind who showed true dedication and loyalty to none other than myself. I would continue to take credit for the perceived good in my life while blaming God, or anyone else, for all of the bad stuff. I was so blind and ignorant of the possibilities ahead.

I was almost two years clean when I was released to a treatment center. I decided that this life was appealing, and I learned so much more about myself. I decided to get a sponsor, homegroup, work steps, and all that fun stuff. Eventually, I got a job. I was offered a position to help open a treatment center, and I really liked it. I always enjoyed learning new things and being a part of something bigger than myself. My pride and ego were getting stroked for being involved in such a great project.

I enjoyed being part of an organization that cared and wanted to help individuals like me. I worked really hard and enjoyed my job very much. That said, the boundaries began to blur between my work and my recovery. Eventually, I was laid off from this position due to a tax-related issue. I was now unemployed and couldn't receive unemployment because I got paid under the table at my previous job and had been in prison.

I was clean for a substantial amount of time, but I had not done all the necessary work on myself to stand firmly grounded when the storm came. I lost my job and didn't have a place to live, so I moved in with my sponsor. I felt horrible and decided that God had it out for me again. What was with this God, always kicking me when I was down? I couldn't understand why all these things were happening to me.

I relapsed, got honest, and tried to get back on the horse. I was given a second chance at my place of employment. Shortly afterwards, my sponsor got very sick and passed away suddenly from untreated hepatitis C. I was asked to move out of his place. I got outraged and resentful. I had no vehicle, sponsor, or job and was now homeless, unable to ask for help. As always, I resorted to my old ways during the raging storm. Blaming God, and everyone else for my problems, never able to admit or even see how I played a part in all of this. I fell into my victim role, and 'poor me' led to 'pour me another drink.'

I bounced in and out of treatment centers and halfway houses for about two years. I continued to worry about how others perceived me. I later learned that how I think others view me is not based on facts but on feelings of inadequacy and low self-worth. I allowed my emotions to dictate my decisions for so many years. I can now see things from a different lens. I can hold myself accountable and assume responsibility for my choices and actions.

I've realized that my thoughts and feelings will lead me astray. I can no longer act on impulse based on a feeling, emotion, or perception. The time I spent in one treatment center after another had been more beneficial than I've ever cared to admit. I've had the privilege of working with some of the best in the field. I've learned so much about myself and how I think about the past. I have gained incredible insight, and I now perceive these times as gifts I've received along the way, even my relapses!

So, this now brings me to my last run, if you will. I had left another halfway house unsuccessfully. I was now in New Castle, PA. I wrote earlier about the monotony of treatment and the rules I was expected to follow. I still don't do well in this regard, but I can say that it keeps getting better.

I moved into a recovery house and was assigned a sponsor. I went to the home group sessions, worked the steps, and worshipped. I had a great job in construction. As a matter of fact, a homegroup member saw my progress and decided to help me. He is the one who helped me find a recovery house to move into. He helped me find a job and ensured I had all I needed. We developed a genuine friendship that is still going strong today!

The pandemic came, and everything was shutting down. The meetings stopped, and I lost my job. My housemates got kicked out because they were using drugs... what a mess. I talked to my sponsor but couldn't shake the feelings I had.

I did not want to do the work to stay clean. I felt like it was the beginning of the zombie apocalypse. My friend and fellow homegroup member, Justin, had relapsed... as did the rest of the house. It was tough because I didn't know how to help him.

Losing him to his addiction threw me into a tailspin. It made me want to start using again. But I couldn't pick up the phone and call anyone because I was afraid of how they would view me. So many people were so proud of how good I was doing. They didn't know I was struggling because I'm not an easy read. I may have a smile and laugh on the outside but be dying inside. The shameful part was my inability to trust or let people in.

I decided to call my friend, Justin. I knew he was from the area and was already getting high. It's funny how easy it is to call someone and say, "Hey, make the call. I'm on the way over and have plenty of cash."

Why couldn't that call be to someone who would guide me and help me through my pain? First of all, I believe that Justin couldn't tell me no because I had his card. Secondly, I knew he was probably broke and needed me. I also knew that he would not judge me or tell me something I didn't want to hear.

Choosing who to call was as natural as breathing air. I decided to call someone who understood me and would help me instead of calling someone that would bring more pain in the long run. I decided on the path of least resistance. All I wanted was instant relief from my pain. So, I consciously decided to 'pick up' with him. Once I did what I did, there would be no stopping me.

I called my sponsor and confessed to him that I had started using again. I also told him I wanted to stop and meant it this time. I was lying to myself yet again. I couldn't stop. At that point, I had become powerless. The compulsion controlled me. I wanted to make money again. In my experience, the only way for someone to get high is to start robbing people or start selling again. Within a week, I had my own apartment and dedicated myself, once again, to destroying everything.

I became a supplier again. I decided it was time to play a high-stakes game. If I was going to play, I would place the biggest bet ever. The high stakes table had a seat reserved for me. They knew it was only a matter of time before I would show my face again.

I learned a few things over the years. I realized I was really good at reading and manipulating people. I invited some dealers over and had enough money to buy them out. Eventually, they could no longer keep up with my supply and demand. They had no choice but to bring in their higher-ups. I finally cut out the middleman. This is a business and, within a month, had enough clientele to move up the ladder. Now the dealers I once had were buying from me.

My friend got out of detox and ended up homeless. I decided to help him out. I didn't intend to hurt him, but I enabled him by allowing him to move in. I used him to run my operation. I degraded myself and everyone who came into contact with me. When I am under the influence, I live at an animalistic level. It's like a Dr. Jekyll / Mr. Hyde kind of thing. I will stop at nothing to move up the ladder and go through anyone who tries to stop me.

I was now using ten times more than before to get the same effect. Recovery had blown my high. I could no longer plead ignorance and knew there was a better way. I continued to use substances, tried to numb all the pain, and ignored what I had learned over the years.

I had no intention of returning to the fellowship or another treatment center. When my friend decided to seek help, it was too late. He pleaded with me to go with him. With the deepest regret in my heart, I turned down the opportunity. I was not ready.

Rarely is a person like me prepared to change anything unless it gets changed for him.

I watched him leave for treatment, and I was angry. I felt I needed him there to help me and I couldn't trust anyone else. I had hundreds of stops made at my house on any given day. People stopped by, getting what they needed, getting high, women working for me, and firearms moving in and out of this place.

One day, I received a letter from a close friend, who informed me that he missed me and was doing really well. I knew his light had returned. I wallowed in self-pity and cried for the first time in years. I had tears of joy that my brother was safe, but I saw no way out of this for myself. My pride and ego were not allowing me to make a rational decision. I was going to die like this and was ok with it.

This was P.R.I.D.E... Primary Reason I Die Early.

I was making a delivery one day and got pulled over. I was arrested for possession of heroin and a few bags of cocaine. I woke up in jail after a nine-day high. I was screwed now! Not a single person could get me out of this one. I was lying on the cot in the processing area and slept peacefully for the first time in months. Finally, it was all over, and part of me was grateful for a brief second.

I got arraigned and called my father to post my bond. He said, "No! Absolutely not!" and hung up on me. The enabling was over, and I was stuck. I didn't know any other numbers by heart, and the police had my phone. I went back to my cell, and for the first time, I didn't try to come up with a plan. I was beaten down and exhausted. The fight was finally over, and I had no way out. I closed my eyes and went to sleep.

I awoke to an officer screaming at me; what a surprise. I was confused, though. It was my first time in this particular jail, and they did things differently. I was being released. My bond was paid in full. What was going on? I haven't a clue. Was I dreaming or hallucinating again? I asked one question, "Who paid my bond?" Molly and Maggy posted my bond. Wow, my girls had come for me, and my mind instantly went back into savage mode.

Maggie came to the rescue. She was out on bond herself and couldn't sign for me, so Molly did. I was convinced that these women truly loved me and missed me. So badly, I wanted to believe that people in this world did love me, but I knew better. They needed me, and I've learned that people living this lifestyle always have ulterior motives.

As soon as I got in the car, they handed me a pipe stuffed to the rim and 2 syringes fully loaded. They knew I would be sicker than a dog. I loved these women at that moment. Maybe they didn't love me, but they loved what I was able to do for them, and that was enough. So, I settled for what I could get. It's crazy what I tried to hold onto even when I knew, in my heart, it was a lie.

A few days later, I was robbed while I was sleeping. This broke my heart. I loved these women despite knowing what they were capable of. In me, the white knight was still trying to save someone who didn't want to be saved. One of the many cycles not easily broken. I will also admit that I didn't treat these women, or anyone else, with respect. They were probably justified in what they did. After all, we chose to play the game and had to accept the outcome. I often wonder how people really felt about me, yet I know it doesn't matter.

I owed a lot of money to several dealers, even more than before, because the police took the drugs I had on me, and my girls sold them to post my bail.

I've been told I could sell ice to an Eskimo, and I convinced them I could get it for them in just a few hours. Despite the trust issues, they consented, knowing I was fully capable of delivering on my promise.

I needed a new phone because I can't make money without a phone. My life of chaos continued as I robbed Peter to pay Paul. The truth is, I didn't care about paying my debts off anymore. I wanted to die and knew I would eventually be going back to prison. I had excellent 'street credit' and a large customer base. I had so much power over people. People would fight to clean my house, do my laundry, and bring me cartons of smokes and stolen goods. I had a stack of bank cards...credit cards, debit cards, and Reliacards... you name it, I probably had it.

People were robbing other drug dealers in my area and bringing me their supplies. One drug dealer was killed just a block away from my home. The police were watching me, pulling people over on my street while I stood at the back door with a gun and samurai sword waiting for whoever was coming next. It could be the drug task force, the attorney general's office, the Drug Enforcement Agency, or the dealers wanting revenge. I was paranoid and convinced that someone was always on their way.

My paranoid psychosis was more intense than I had ever experienced. People were now afraid to come to me for what they needed. I was bat shit crazy! I held a friend against the wall with a knife to his throat because I thought he was trying to set me up. I had lost touch with reality. Everyone had motives. Either tried to set me up or rob me. I was losing my mind. I couldn't sleep and was up for weeks at a time. I felt isolated and alone. I was restless, irritable, and unhappy. What happened next will be a significant contributing factor to my PTSD. It still plagues me to this day.

I had controlled so many people, yet I had never felt so alone in my entire life. Nobody was to be trusted... least of all me. Eventually, a roommate of mine set me up. After being awake for weeks, I was lying in my bed, tucked in with a new woman. They tried for days to get me to sleep. I was so weak that I couldn't stand without help. I looked like one of the blow-up mascots that wave in the wind on car lots. My mind had shut down, and my body was trying to follow. Shocked, I awoke to a man standing over me. The woman beside me screamed in terror as a hammer swung at my face. I have no idea how he missed me. I can only remember rolling off the bed as I struggled to avoid his swings. Unfortunately, this was not one of my dreams.

I couldn't believe this was really happening. I was in a state of shock. We fought each other until we were both physically exhausted. I dove for my gun as he screamed, "Just give me the cash and the dope!". As I reached for my gun, I got smashed in the back of the head with a hammer! As I stood up, he punched me with fierce determination to win this battle. This intruder needed to die because it would be him or me, and I saw no other way.

As I struggled to get to my feet, I noticed blood everywhere. It was saturating my new carpet, in my eyes and all over the floor. The hammer was still in his hand when I realized I was bleeding out. I saw the next swing coming and grabbed his wrist before he made the connection. Physically drained, mentally depleted, and spiritually dead, I thought, 'why isn't anyone helping me?' My roommates just stood there, watching in the background.

I was wearing what was now a crimson red hooded sweatshirt, and I had a coppery taste in my mouth. I saw the fear in the burglar's eyes as I stared into his soul. He dropped the hammer, and it hit the floor. I collapsed. I was physically drained and had lost so much blood. I followed his eyes as they moved to my wallet lying on the floor. As he leaned over to take it, I hit him with all I had left. It felt like the slowest, weakest punch I had ever thrown! I punched him in slow motion as he turned and unlocked the door. He jumped off of my porch and got into a white car.

I thought to myself, this is what my life has come to. I was almost murdered in front of two people living with me rent-free. In exchange for their services, I supplied their habits, yet neither of them had any loyalty to me. They wouldn't help me.

I wanted everyone out of my house, but I couldn't be alone. Even though I had felt alone and hopeless for months, I still needed to be validated. I still needed help and human companionship... no matter how wretched the humans were.

One roommate cleaned me up a bit, and the other started cooking my next few spoonfuls of heroin. We treated my wound with a piece of duct tape. People started showing up with weapons, angry that I was assaulted. Apparently, people did need me and did want to protect me... or so it seemed.

43

In reality, they were protecting their investments and the place of operation that paid them. I now had people at both doors armed and waiting. We needed to rebound and get the money right so I could open another 'shop.' This one was compromised. I still had an ample supply and all my cash. I was almost murdered for a wallet full of cards, which I canceled immediately.

There would be no trip to the hospital, no call for an ambulance, and definitely no call to law enforcement. These people would ask questions, and I could give no answers. Finally, I felt safe enough to rest, if only for a little while. I laid down in my bed with both doors guarded and another woman in my bed as I drifted off.

I got woken up by a new high-stakes player. This man was new to me, yet he admitted he was a fan of my loyalty and dedication to his organization. He and I spoke for quite a while in the presence of his two younger brothers. They wanted to know what my next move was going to be. We discussed who was to be trusted and who was not. Eventually, the leader asked me to distribute his products in mass quantity. I was given more drugs and weapons than I had any business having.

I had already decided I wanted out, but I played his game with one objective in mind. I would need all he had to offer to start a new life. So, I deceived this man into giving me more than he originally intended. I convinced him that his brothers would be allowed to stop and check on me whenever they wanted. I even gave them a key to my house... or so they thought. I took a gamble, assuming they would not check to see if the key fit the lock. Actually, the key belonged to a house several blocks away.

I had played my cards right and got the jackpot. I was now an expert poker player. The moment these men left, I had a few trusted people at my place packing. We were out of the house with my most prized belongings in less than an hour. I left a lot behind to make people think I was still living there. I drove a few hours away and picked up a few women I had known from long ago. Their dealer needed a new plug, and I had what he was looking for. I thought, what the heck? I needed the cash and wanted to see my girls. It was a win-win.

I never had a driver's license. I always got a car from a fellow addict. It was a new Subaru this time, and that car was fast! I made the trip in half the time, filling my need for speed and adrenaline. My girls and I were partying in the car with mass quantities of illegal substances and weapons. They decided they wanted milkshakes. Milkshakes while smoking crack cocaine?! I found that strange, but I pulled into a Sheetz just up the street. Some state police were in the parking lot, and I was lying back in my seat, asking myself, where the hell did these girls go? What on earth was taking them so long? I almost left them behind but couldn't bring myself to do it. Curiosity got the best of me, so I proceeded to stroll into Sheet's and get my own milkshake. What happened next would change my life and how I viewed things forever.

I saw someone who looked familiar and then I heard her voice. The shame, embarrassment, and broken state I was in had never seemed so relevant. Mandy, a supervisor I knew from the treatment center, was standing there looking at me through glassy, tear-filled eyes. I saw the pain and general disgust on her face as she looked at me. She could tell I was broken. I was covered in track marks, sixty pounds lighter than usual, two blood clots in my leg, and black tar heroin seeping out of a fresh wound on my arm. She told me to call her the next day, and she would get me a bed in detox and treatment. I knew I wouldn't follow through, so I asked her to call me. I still had no intention of going into treatment again.

We got back in the car, and off we went. The ride would change my life forever. We were going 120 miles per hour on Route 279, and I couldn't shake the feeling of shame that I had. No amount of drugs I consumed would kill the pain.

I smoked and shot enough drugs on that ride to wipe out an entire family twice. The pain, shame, fear, and everything else I was experiencing would not go away. I felt like that for the next 20 hours. I was suicidal and decided to isolate myself in a bathroom. Mandy, a friend true to her word, called just in time. She said, "Are you ready?" and the word "Yes" came out of my mouth.

I realized the drugs weren't the solution to my problems. In fact, they stopped working. I had no veins left. I was dehydrated, and I cried for hours. I was at a fork in the road. My choices were to leave this world for good or find a new way to live. Less than three minutes later, I was called by someone in admissions, and we discussed my treatment options. I didn't need a ride. I wanted to take myself there to tie up a few loose ends first.

I woke up in treatment a few days later, not knowing what had happened. I stumbled out of a room that was so very familiar to me. I had been here before and knew half of the staff members. An ex-girlfriend of mine walked in, and she looked really good. At this point, she was two years clean and working there herself. I thought I was hallucinating or dreaming again.

I crawled back into bed and slept for two more days. One of my best friends was tucking me in as I thrashed around and spasmed in pain. Luke was here getting help too, or was it all a dream? I woke several times, looking around for my phone, drugs, and gun. I flipped my mattress over in a state of panic several times, looking for anything that could take the pain away. I found nothing.

The battle raged on in my mind, heart, and soul for weeks to come. I wanted to run so badly, and the gravitational pull was strong. My people were there for me, though. Luke, and three of my best customers, were in treatment with me. All the people who worked here knew me and how I operated as an addict. I had genuine love and support for the first time ever. They would not allow me to leave, even if it meant physically holding me down.

A man I knew from a prior visit was starting a class called Psalm 91, from a book by Peggy Joyce Ruth. I didn't want to attend because I was not religious, but something called me to him. Or, perhaps it was because I didn't want to sit with the larger group. All I know is I was right where I was meant to be.

I don't understand why I've survived as long as I have. I have overdosed more than twenty times. I've been in more car accidents than I care to admit. I drove through a restaurant in downtown Pittsburgh. I've been stabbed 6 times, shot at, chased from state to state by vicious people, contemplated suicide, and hospitalized more times than I can count. I've made it through unbearable, unexplainable situations. The fact that I'm not doing life in prison or dead is a miracle.

My pride and ego were my real enemies, nearly killing me. Today I view my life as a gift. I know, in my heart, that I had nothing to do with all the blessings I've received, good or bad, over the years. I have learned that not everything should be perceived as good or bad. Sometimes things just are what they are, and we have to wait to receive the gifts given to us! Patience is something I'm still working on. I've learned to use my time and my support system wisely.

I was once told a story that I want to share with you because it changed how I perceive the world today.

A small Chinese man lived in a village. He was the village Elder. He had one son, no wife, and a plow horse, which was the only way he would make any money. They lived in a small cottage made of straw and clay. One day the Elder woke to find his fence broken and his horse gone. A local villager from around the way came by and said to this Elder, "That's horrible. Whatever shall you do now?" The old man responded, "I don't know if it's good or bad; maybe it just is." The locals thought the Elder must be losing it. The very next day, the Elder woke to a stampede of horses running through his property!

His son was trampled by the arrival of all these horses, and both of his legs were now broken. The local returned and said to the Elder, "That's horrible what happened to your son. What will you do now?" The Elder replied, "I do not know that it is good or bad; maybe it just is." The next day the General of the local army arrived in the village and took all the children away to train for war. The Elder stayed in his house of straw and clay, nursing his son back to health while his horses plowed for the village!

This is so powerful and taught me so much! Sometimes I need to be patient and try not to get so angry over the small things. Will these small things be remembered a day, a week, a month from now, anyway? I learned that sometimes things aren't necessarily good or bad; maybe they just are. I also learned that I may have something on the horizon that is much more incredible than anything I could ever imagine! However, I'm just not able to see it!

To this day, I am still not a religious person. I believe wholeheartedly in the power of prayer, nonetheless. I can feel it and know that it is real. Especially when it's done sincerely from the heart. I can only speculate why I am here sharing my story with you. You see, today, I have found a third purpose in life: to help as many people overcome their demons as possible.

As sure as I know the sky is blue, I am certain I have a higher power watching over me. One that has had my back for as long as I can remember. I remember wanting to leave my first rehab. It was the first time I had ever gone through a severe withdrawal, and I wanted to sign out and run. As I sat in a gazebo, contemplating my departure, I sensed a moment of peace I would later know as a spiritual experience. The snow began to fall, and it was the first time I noticed how perfect a snowflake was. As a kid, I made them out of paper. But in that moment, I was personally witnessing the perfection and beauty of something so small. I know today that my higher power was trying to calm my inner storm.

I have had several experiences like this over the years, yet I was blind and unable to recognize them for what they were. The time in the horse barn, the time in bed deciding whether I should stay behind or not run. The time that Jiminy Cricket told me, "You're doing wrong, stop it!". I could go on for days about everything I missed when I was rushing to destroy everyone's life... including my own.

Today I see the beauty in most things. I have learned that I will find what I am looking for, and the law of attraction does, in fact, exist, just like in the book The Secret. My creativity and imagination are beautiful assets now. I developed it as a coping mechanism. My dedication to meditation has helped me tremendously. So much of my life directly resulted from my trauma and PTSD. As I've said before, my perceptions of everything terrible may not be accurate. I have learned to dig deep and seek meaning in all things.

I view my mother's death very differently now. The man I found dead saved my life, and I realize now that he was sick. I have to assume responsibility for my part in all of this. I sold that man and my mother drugs, enabling their addictions. I know today that my mother no longer suffers. She is finally at peace and able to rest. She looks down on me... proud of her son. I sleep better at night, knowing these things to be true. She no longer suffers, and neither do I. We are free today, and that is such a blessing. I am not cured. I still have episodes, but they are few and far between now. Most of my trauma stems from my life, my actions, and what I've seen over the years. It is much better than it used to be and gets better every day!

I am honored and thrilled to have a sense of purpose that is quite rewarding. There is no denying that a higher power is at work. How else would I still be here? Today I no longer take all the credit. I give thanks and gratitude for my life. I will cherish it to the best of my ability and never take it for granted.

When we choose to help each other, we can accomplish anything. People who have overcome their own demons have given me a new set of lenses to look through! Thank you, predecessors!

Think of a playing card for a second. Each card is frail, slender, and easily torn by itself. But, together, it makes a sturdy deck of cards, which is not easily torn apart. I need the people in my life who want to see me make a difference and push me to become the best version of myself.

I've learned that the people who do not contribute to my recovery or personal growth need to go, even if they are family. I've learned I have all the love I could imagine if I'm willing to ask for it.

As I write this, it's just a few short days before Christmas, and I get to fulfill one of my most prolonged desires, to become a published author. I have people in my corner who believe in me and continue to help me recover. They encourage me to do the right thing.

I am very grateful to have had this opportunity to share my experience, strength, and hope with you!

H.O.P.E. = Help Open People's Eyes!

I try to remember that as I continue to better myself and the people around me. Thank you so very much, Kathleen Sarro, for this combined effort and collaboration so that we can bring hope to those who need it. You have always believed in me and pushed me to write this story. I appreciate the love and generosity of you and your family!

Sincerely yours,

 John

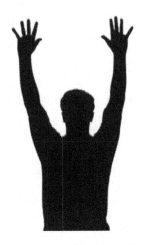

CHAPTER TWO

If I Can Do It, You Can Too!

By Kalena

"The only person you are destined to become is the person you decide to be."

– Ralph Waldo Emerson

My name is Kalena, and I'm an addict.

I've been clean from heroin since November 8, 2015, and sober from alcohol since September 26, 2019. My story starts out quite different from most addicts and alcoholics. For one, I am not a product of my environment. My parents handed me the world on a silver platter from an early age. I was given the gift of a blessed life.

From pre-school through eighth grade, I attended a private school. I was an only child, and my parents ensured I always had the best of everything. By everything, I mean clothes, shoes, a sports car with a big red bow on it for my 'Sweet 16', European vacations, and prom gowns from Paris. They made certain college was paid for, and I could come out free of debt. My life was perfect.

In 2004, I got an opportunity to become a flight attendant, and while this life may appear glamorous to most, it is a lonely one. I found great comfort in alcohol. It helped me relax in foreign locations and constantly surrounded by people I didn't know.

In 2006, I gave it up to move home after trying to take my own life by swallowing a bottle of Xanax. I discovered that my longtime boyfriend had been secretly videotaping very private parts of my life. It was then I decided to tell my parents a secret I had been hiding since 1999. At the age of 15, I was raped by a classmate. After that, I was never the same.

In January of 2008, I met my first husband. He was in the military and said all the right things when I needed to hear them the most. Just two months later, we married. He was deployed to Iraq on May 9, 2008, and on May 18, 2008, I got a phone call saying I was pregnant with our first child. I was diligent about remaining sober throughout my pregnancy and never drank a sip of alcohol or consumed any type of medication that could possibly harm my child.

My daughter was born prematurely in December 2008, and my whole life changed. At the time, my marriage was a loveless marriage of convenience and alcohol again became my companion. After a few years of physical, mental, and emotional abuse, we divorced. That's when drinking became my priority. I was home alone with a baby and overwhelmed with fear of what was next.

Fast forward to June of 2011 when I met my second husband. We married in December 2012, and I don't think I was sober for even one day of our marriage. I was not a wife to him, but I always made sure I was a mother to my daughter. Even as a functioning alcoholic, my daughter always came first.

In July of 2014, I found out my husband was having an affair. It killed me, but I knew it was my fault. I was not a wife to him. I was just an alcoholic with whom he resided, and in August of 2014, he left.

My drinking took a significant turn for the worse, and my father did everything he could to help me. He took me to meetings out of the county, so I didn't have to see people I knew. He kept me busy with activities, and my mother never stopped loving me. They were always there to pick up the pieces of their shattered daughter.

Finally, in January of 2015, they had enough and had me arrested and put into an institution. However, as an alcoholic, I was the master of manipulation and manipulated the nurses and psychiatrists to let me go.

I think I was sober for 16 days before I drank again. Shortly after my release from the institution, I reconnected with an individual who used to work for me. He manipulated me in the same ways I used to manipulate everyone in my life. You think I would have known what he was doing, but I didn't. This is where everything took a turn for the worse.

In August 2015, I married my third husband—the heroin addict and master manipulator. He was always disappearing for days at a time, taking my bank card with him. I noticed thousands of dollars missing, but I thought he could be helped. That was until he asked me if I wanted to try heroin too. Without any hesitation, my curiosity was piqued, so I said yes.

One time was all it took, and I was caught up in a whole new world. I lost jobs, I lost my home, I lost my car, and I lost myself. But one thing I never lost was my daughter. She meant more to me than anything. So, in November 2015, when I awoke in a bathtub filled with cold water with my clothes soaked after an overdose, I decided to get help. I entered a program through Narcotics Anonymous and I've been clean from heroin since November 8th, 2015. Since then, I've never looked back.

In 2016, my husband was sentenced to prison, yet again, so I filed for divorce and came crawling home to my parents, who took me in yet again. My parents always tried so hard to save me, but all the love in the world cannot save a person with an addiction to alcohol until they want to be saved. Finally, in November 2017, my parents had enough of my alcohol addiction and threw me out. My daughter remained at their home because I truly had nowhere to go.

They had enough of the physical, mental, and emotional abuse I put them through after all those years, and it was then they chose to move on in life without me. This killed me. I began to drown my sorrows with more alcohol than I ever drank before, but it didn't work. In December they had me arrested again and placed back into an institution. This time, I genuinely tried to give it a go. I stayed there for five days, and when I was released, I had nowhere to go, no parents, no money, and no daughter. My parents declared me as an unfit mother and used the court system to get custody.

I was hopeless and lost. Within 30 days, I lived with a drug dealer and drank myself into oblivion every single day for the next year and a half. I wanted my daughter back, but I realized that they didn't take her from me; I lost her due to my alcoholism. No amount of alcohol could take away the broken and empty feeling I felt after losing her. My daughter was the only thing in my life that ever made sense. She was my greatest gift, but now she was gone too.

The dealer I was living with was very abusive. The more I drank, the less I felt. In that year and a half, I suffered 17 broken bones, four concussions, a five-day coma, and I was beaten within an inch of my life… twice. In March 2019, he was finally taken to prison, and I was free from him, but not from my alcoholism. In fact, ironically, it got worse.

Eventually, I received a friend request on Facebook from a man I never met. Something about him made me want to meet him. Little did I know, this man would save my life. I pressed accept. He asked me to go to a local amusement park for a date, and I said yes.

However, I knew my alcoholism would prevent anyone from wanting to get to know the real me, so I tried desperately to stop on my own. Let's just say that was a huge mistake. Alcohol withdrawal is far worse than heroin withdrawal and is never something you should try to do alone.

The day we were supposed to meet, I suffered a grand mal seizure from withdrawal. He called and texted all day that day, wondering what happened to me, but I was in the hospital with no phone. When I got out, I had to drink to 'be well.' I couldn't tell him the truth.

One day he asked me out to dinner, and we went out on our first date.

At this point, I was functioning, and unless you knew me personally, you would have never known I was an alcoholic. After our date, we went back to his place to have a few drinks. We talked for hours getting to know each other. When it was time to go, he said to me, "I don't want you to leave", so I never did.

For the next few months, he noticed my alcoholism but loved me anyway. He loved me through my pain, my suffering, and my heartbreak. He saw something in me I never saw in myself. On July 4, 2019, underneath the fireworks, he asked me to be his wife.

The word 'yes' had never been said so easily or with such certainty, but I knew I could not go on this way. At this point, I was consuming over five boxes of wine, equivalent to 30 gallons, every single day.

My body was failing me, and I wanted a better life. I wanted this marriage to work. I wanted my parents to be proud of me. I wanted my daughter back. I didn't want to be the person people would cross the street to avoid anymore. So, I realized it was time to change, so I took a chance and decided to go to rehab. For the first time, on September 26th, I woke up sober. I haven't had a drink since then.

On October 26, 2019, my 30th day sober, I married my fourth and final husband, the one who loved me back to life was now my husband! Then, after a year of sobriety, I started the journey of regaining custody of my daughter. And to this day, I am still battling my parents in court who refuse to give her back to me.

Throughout these last three years, I have done everything I can to try to get back into my parents' lives. But, unfortunately, forgiving me is something they refuse to do. When we were ordered to court-appointed counseling, I sat in horror with tears running slowly down my face as my father said, 'We want nothing to do with her.' I was crushed, but I didn't drink.

Every holiday, Mother's Day, Father's Day, and every birthday, I find a way to send something to them to let them know their daughter is still here and loves them unconditionally. Making amends in recovery is not easy and not everyone is willing to accept you, but when it comes to my parents, I will never give up. I will show them I am no longer the addict or alcoholic who destroyed and broke their hearts. I was a person who was lost and held captive to an addiction that had more power over me than I had over myself. I will have my parents back one day, even if it takes me to my last breath. Perhaps even more importantly, I will get my daughter back. No child deserves to be kept from their mother. So, no matter how hard it gets, I will never give up.

So that is who I was and where I came from.

Today, I am over six years clean and almost three years sober. Today, I am the best mother I can be to my daughter while sharing custody until the battle is over. I am a stepmother to two wonderful sons. I am a wife to a man who never gave up on me. I have a budding career as a healthcare recruiter at a company that I adore.

Today, I have a small circle of great friends. Today, I am one of the most sought-after sponsors in recovery. Today, I am a grateful and recovering addict and alcoholic named Kalena.

If you are struggling with addiction or alcoholism, please know that if I can recover, you can too!

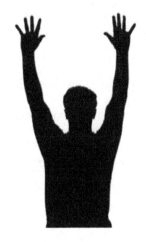

CHAPTER THREE

By God's Grace

By Earl

"When everything seems to be going against you, remember that the airplane takes off against the wind, not with it."

– Henry Ford

Life has been good to me now, probably better than anyone with addiction issues. I have been blessed with the opportunity to enter a Medication-Assisted Treatment (MAT) program. I had many people at the clinic who listened to me and helped me better understand myself. With the help of so many caring, non-judgmental, beautiful people, I learned that I needed to rewire my brain and change the way I think. I thank all of them for believing in me, even when I did not believe in myself.

The people who work at this MAT set aside all my aggravation and bullheadedness and taught me new ways to cope with stress.

At one point, I thought help wasn't possible. They proved to me otherwise. Being healthy is now part of my day-to-day routine. I want to thank everyone at the MAT Program for never giving up on me and continuing to believe in me. Thank you.

Hello friends, my name is Earl. My addiction always had its price, and I learned this the hard way, as many do. For many years, I never thought I had a problem. I thought my life was normal. For a long time, I refused to admit that I had a problem. Until, one day, I decided I wanted to kill myself.

I was sick and tired of being sick and tired if that makes any sense at all. Deep down, I was crying for help, and I didn't know what to do or how to get the help I needed. I remember it was August 2010, and I was living in a trailer in Hermitage, Pennsylvania. It was a scorching summer, and I had just come home from the Welfare office.

It was sweltering inside my trailer. I didn't have any air conditioning. Just a small fan. I sat down, stared at the Welfare book in my hand, and started crying. At the time, I was very dope sick and a little suicidal. The fan was blowing the pages of the booklet open, and the page that opened caught my interest. "You Can Stop Addiction." There was a phone number and I thought, "Maybe this is a sign." I had been praying like hell to be relieved from the horrible pain.

I made the call, and the person I spoke to told me about the MAT program that was close by. So, I called the clinic, and they said I could start the next morning. They told me to hang in there and assured me that my life would get better soon. I just needed to be strong right now.

The following day, I took my very first dose of Methadone. At the time, I did not even know what Methadone was. I said out loud, "There is a God!". From that day on, my life changed in ways I could never have imagined, and it was for all the better.

I can't really explain it, but for some odd reason, Methadone made me help myself, and it helped me change the person I was. Initially, I was afraid that it would not work because it seemed like everything in my life didn't work... so why would this? This was different. I wanted to help myself and rise above my past.

By God's grace and, with the help of Methadone, I stopped drinking, stayed out of neighborhoods where I got the dope, and stayed away from negative people. I don't know what happened, but it changed me forever. I feel so much better being drugfree. I really don't think I could have done what I have without the MAT treatment.

I continue to enjoy all the wonderful support from my counselor, support groups, and nurses. There are so many kind hearts that have helped me on my drug free journey. Most addicts cannot do it on their own. They need help in various ways, including the support of people who really want to help, and will go out of their way to make change happen.

The Medication-Assisted Treatment keeps me in line. Counseling, support groups, and urine screens make me responsible. I found that I need structure and accountability. So, it's been over 10 years, and I am proud to say that, since that call to MAT, I have never looked back or gone out to the streets.

The structure is what is needed so that the brain can get rewired. Miracles can happen. I am sure of this because I am one of them.

If you are willing to fight and do the work, the staff will fight for you. They will make sure you get what you need so change can happen. It's almost like a car. Addicts need to break down and get rebuilt. Change can happen when you change the way you think, develop strong coping skills, and learn better ways to deal with stress. Sometimes, things need to be torn down and rebuilt.

The people at the clinic are there to help us fix ourselves. How can we maintain this 'new' person so that the new healthy person is now the new normal? I am not ashamed to say that I got the help I needed to learn how to do and be better because I was not able to do this on my own. I did not understand why I was the way I was. I needed to be educated and counseled on why and how to change. I learned that once I developed better ways to cope with stress, I also needed to practice the techniques so I could stay healthy. I needed to be taught. I needed people to care for and believe in me. This is what I got from MAT. It has worked miracles on me.

I can say I love my life now, and I love the person I am! That day, in August 2010, my life changed forever! I have been at the same job for 10 years now. I have a happy, strong family and am grateful for everything.

I go once a week; I have slowly lowered my dose over the years. Will I ever leave Methadone? I don't know. All I do know is I am a changed human being. I work hard. I am responsible. I love God and my fellow mankind. I am kind and drug free. I obey the law, and I'm never in trouble.

One day, I may taper back and get completely off of Methadone. That said, I also know the person I was back then. I like the new me better, and if it means doing what I am doing, I am okay with that.

Before anyone forms an opinion, I am here to tell you, "Do whatever works." I am not saying my methods will work for everyone. I am just saying active addicts are desperate and sick people, and the last thing anyone should do is to judge or be critical, regardless of their treatment of choice.

I go to the clinic once a week, and when I leave there, it almost feels like I am leaving church. I feel great now! I can visit people at any time who will listen to me, care about me, and help me if I need it. I know that there are so many more good people in the world. I am grateful to the staff, and I feel that there is a spot in Heaven for all of them. From the bottom of my heart,

Thank you!

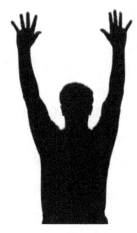

CHAPTER FOUR

Connecting With God

By Mr. V

"Never underestimate a recovering addict. We fight for our lives every day in ways most people will never understand."

– Unknown

For the past 24 hours, I have found myself wondering what I should write about when it comes to this crazy thing called addiction. Then I realized that I am actually excited to write this, now 12 years later. So, where do I start?

I'm sitting in rehab at age 34 surrounded by people about ten years younger than me. Their stories all made sense and sadly, all of them were tragic. Some of the stories I heard included "my uncle molested me at the age of five", "my babysitter got me at 12", "my mother was a junkie", "I started to shoot up with my parents", and "my stepdad beat me". I can see why many people struggle like hell to get out of their addiction.

My story isn't so clear cut. I didn't have any childhood traumas, per se, and I had decent, good parents. We grew up poor, but we always had food, lived in a decent home, and we were never cold. Although, I had a few distant aunts and uncles that may have had drinking issues. So, I guess I can start there.

When I was around 12 years old, I started to steal beer from the fridge. Over time, I drank more and more. By the age of 18, I was a hard-core alcoholic. I probably drank 12 to 20 beers a day. At a fairly young age, I ended up getting my license taken away. I really didn't care though. I was young and could ride my bike anywhere I wanted to go. Sometimes, I'd ride 100's of miles a week.

In 12th grade, drinking became my priority, so I decided to quit school. At the time, a family member came to visit, and asked me if I wanted to go on a 'trip'. I knew to stay away from the so-called 'physically addicting' drugs but I thought I could experiment with some others as long as they didn't interfere with my drinking. I thought it would be cool to try something new.

We decided to go down to the river, and I was given five dots of double-dipped blotter acid. I thought it might be too much to do all five at once, so I only took two of them. The next thing I remember, I was standing in a circle, laughing with about seven people at the camp. Little did I know, I was getting ready to black out.

The next memory I had was running with people on the edge of a cliff until I blacked out again. When I came to, I was swinging on a rope over the river Then… I blacked out again.

When I regained consciousness, it was pitch black and I was under the biggest, whitest moon I had ever seen. We climbed into a canoe and took off. As we approached what I thought was a waterfall, we decided to stop at a dock. I was a little more conscious now; I could tell that the waterfall was just a bend in the water.

It was my turn to exit the boat. Wait! Something is wrong! I feel panic rising in me. I can't get out of the boat. I am dragging my legs… as if my legs were dead. Apparently, I had been sitting cross legged for hours. It turns out that 12 hours had passed but I was only aware of the last 10 minutes.

As the panic and intensity subsided, I began to enjoy the sights as we returned to camp. We built a fire and began to drink again… until I hit on a fat, ugly chick and then throw up.

Suffice it to say, I was forever changed that day… for better or for worse, that's hard to say! That said, there's no doubt I was a man who fell in love with tripping. At the end of my drinking binges, I would do speeders and cocaine. That said, I could always stop before it got the better of me.

In my mid 20's, I moved to Las Vegas. At the time, pot took a back seat, and alcohol and cocaine were my drug of choice because it was cheap… but they nearly took my life.

Eventually, I had my first experience with opiates when a guy from work shared his Percocets. I absolutely loved it! I had abused

68

my body over the years, and now I actually felt great! I felt like I was 18 again! I had endurance and strength. It never even occurred to me that I could become physically addicted to it. At the time, I never took enough to get sick. Just enough to feel great, so I didn't have any issues.

Eventually, the same guy from work gave us Oxycontin. We had no idea what they were when we tried them. They were too strong, so I quit taking them. I began experimenting with methamphetamines, commonly known as 'meth', but I wasn't worried about getting addicted. Five here and five there. Drinking was still my focus. I drank seven days a week, 12 hours a day.

Vegas was killing me, and I knew it. I had to make a choice. I could be a pothead and occasional hard drug user or a drinker. I chose to be a pothead and planned my escape from Vegas.

I still remember the drive back because my car overheated as I was going up the mountains as I drove out of there. But, once I cleared the mountains, it was smooth sailing back to Pennsylvania with my tripping buddies.

Before long, I discovered they had a meth contact, and we would spend our nights at the bar. I was trying hard not to drink, but with the meth, it was becoming more and more difficult to stop. I was broken at the time. I would buy $30 worth of meth and just sit around and build puzzles. After a few months of this, I realized it was time to quit using meth. I was still drinking, but only a fraction of what I used to drink.

In my late 20's, I got my own place and wanted to save money for the first time. I found that I had some motivation and determination. I'd drink a 6-pack here and there, but for the most part, I'd just do pot.

Things were starting to look up. Granted my neighbors were crackheads and I would buy a rock every once in a while. At times, I'd only take 2 hits and walk away. My neighbors could not understand how I could do this. However, I was motivated and looked forward to getting better. Almost zero alcohol, or anything else for that matter, so I was happy with myself.

Then... BAM! A devastating car accident.

I'll spare you some of the gory details. However, it was a head-on collision and I didn't have a license. My sternum, every single rib, and my collar bone were all broken. My liver and esophagus were torn. Both my lungs collapsed. I regained consciousness a few minutes after the impact and found my car jack resting on my chest. I managed to lift it off as riveting pain shot through my body. The pain was worse than I anything I had ever experienced. I was coughing up blood... a lot of blood. I thought I was going to die.

A passerby let me use her phone to call my parents. I told them goodbye, that I was going to die but I would be okay. I kept breathing through the excruciating pain and managed to stay conscious. I remember screaming as I was being cut out of my car and moved to the ambulance. At the same time, the screams didn't seem like they belonged to me because they were fading.

During the ambulance ride, I was fading in and out of consciousness. I would wake up screaming whenever we hit a bump. When I arrived in the emergency room, I begged the doctor to do something to stop the unbearable pain. They had to place a tube in me to inflate my lungs. I was unconscious for the next 48 hours.

I was brought out of my medical coma so my family and friends could say goodbye. Unfortunately, I only have a vague recollection of what was happening to me at the time. After a few days, I came out of the coma and was told it was a miracle that I was alive. As I began the healing journey, I had an epidural patch, a Morphine drip, and a daily dose of Oxycontin and Percocet.

The next several weeks were tough. If I sat still, the pain was bearable, but moving was an entirely different story.

The day before I left the hospital, I sat up too fast and howled in pain. The nurse gave me a shot of Morphine. This was the first time I had gotten comfortable and could nod off a bit.

On the 14th day, I was released and moved in with my mom. I couldn't work for the next 4 months and had, again, lost everything. I lost my home, my car… pretty much everything.

The plan I had set in motion was to better my life. However, on top of the crippling pain, I was also up against two felony charges for death or injury while driving without a license.

Suffice it to say my pride was damaged for the first time since I was 19. Now, after all my drinking and drugging in the past, I had a DUI, a suspended license, I was looking at jail time and living with my mother.

During the first three months, they continued to prescribe a daily dose of Oxycontin and Percocet. For the first month, it kept my pain in check as long as I didn't move. In the second month, the pain was bearable, and I was able to start moving around some.

During the third month, I moved in with my dad because my mother lived in the country, and I had difficulty sustaining myself.

I was still in pain, but compared to the pain I had before, it was manageable. I had a few days of my prescriptions left and went to see the orthopedic surgeon. He was going to send me to physical therapy and, when I asked about more pain meds, his assistant said "a month of Vicodin 10's." His response was, "that stuff is nasty." So, he gave me 30 Darvocet instead.

I didn't know what they were, but I was hoping that they'd work and help me get through the pain I was feeling. I didn't realize at the time that I was labeled a 'pain med seeker'. The labeling started in the hospital. I'd ask for more meds because the pain was unbearable during that horrible time.

A couple of days later, I snorted my last Oxycodone. It was nice. I was able to go on a short hike for the first time since the accident. Unfortunately, the next day I got sick... really sick. My pain level began to shoot through the roof. The next day I learned firsthand what it was like to be 'dope sick' and was fortunate enough to get some Oxycodone from a friend.

For the next few months, I really struggled both mentally and physically. Turns out I had a tear in my pelvis which wasn't diagnosed until four years later. At this point I barely touched alcohol anymore and never had my life controlled by drugs. Yet, I was always treated like an addict.

When I went to a pain management program, I was given Ultram. They told me I had to quit smoking weed if I wanted any more Ultram. I may have done that if it helped with the pain but they didn't. So, I decided to go to the chiropractor and get some Oxycodone.

I quit. I used. I quit. I used. This went on for over five months. I struggled with my addiction and, ultimately lost the battle when I was convicted of causing death or injury. I was sentenced to 90 days of house arrest, three years suspension, and regular drug testing. Smoking pot would be too risky, so I started to snort Oxycodone every day.

Pills were getting way too expensive and harder to find so I found myself stealing change out of unlocked cars to pay for my habit. Before long, it became more logical to snort heroin. Needles were not my preference, but this is when the black tar was cheap and plentiful.

I swear I tried to eat, smoke, and snort the tar, but none of it got me high. In just 18 months, I went from a strong, healthy 29-year-old 'man with a plan' to a crippled, convicted felon banging black tar heroin. I was 31 years old, and was totally okay with dying by the time I decided to stick that needle in my arm.

So... I guess I am at that part of my story that everyone wants to hear about. The part where everything goes to shit.

Well, not so fast!

I ended up working in a kitchen where I had made some significant improvements and decent money. And for anyone that was around in the black tar days, they can testify that this was twice as strong as Oxy 80 and cost 75% less. So, I could support a habit and get high for about $200 a week! But, more importantly,

I could function well, work every day and hang out with my non-junkie friends.

I lived like this for about a year, and of course, there was always underlying depression lingering around. Depression is usually coupled with constant lying and sneaking around, but not for me. I was still in a lot of pain because of the tear in my pelvis, and I felt hopeless about it ever getting repaired. Besides the physical pain, I was also mentally numb. I just felt that working hard and playing by the rules never really got me anywhere. I couldn't drink because if I did, I would throw up. So, ironically, it had been over a year since I had any alcohol. This was a huge win for me!

Then one morning, I read a headline in the paper that said, "Black Tar Heroin Ring Busted in Beaver County" (… or something like that). The article said that they were selling drugs for four years and they were being watched for at least three years. If this is true, why the heck did they allow drugs to flood the streets for years before they busted them?! Many people were killed by those drugs!

Truthfully, I had mixed feelings because I knew I was addicted mentally and physically, but I didn't realize how bad it was. The ritual, the rush of buying the drug, using the needles … I was addicted on so many levels! Once this bust happened, I realized it was time to get clean!

I struggled to give up the booze in the past, but I didn't seem to have many issues getting off most of the drugs. However, trying to get off opiates was an entirely different animal. I had no idea how bad it would be so I got as much Suboxone as possible. Let's just say, the worst was yet to come.

The first few days, I took a lot of sleeping pills, so the withdrawal was not too bad. After the first few days of detoxing, my buddy and I left the house for the first time. We sat in the front yard in the sun, feeling exhausted and tired, but it was doable. I had a chance to stay clean and thought that maybe I would.

Later that night, my buddy called and said he had a contact in Pittsburgh and asked me if I wanted anything. Without hesitation, I gathered all the money I could. If this next page or two had a chapter title, it would be called "Stamp Bags Suck!"! Dope wasn't easy to get anymore. It required rides to the city, waiting around, phone calls, collecting other people's money, and the most important issue... three times the amount of money for the same $20 high as in the past. So, what used to cost me $20 just to feel better and function, was now costing me $60!

My job suffered because I was starting to miss work. My ass was dragging. Thanks to my dad's massive amount of spare change and Suboxone, I was able to keep working and stay semi-functional.

Eventually, I became a dealer and had eight to ten people calling me to put their 'orders' in. I felt that if I could make some deals, I'd cut my costs so I don't get sick and could continue to function throughout the day.

After a few short weeks of this, I was fired from the job I had for 3 years. So, I focused on my new job... getting phone calls, wheeling and dealing all day. Most days, I'd collect $200 -$400. The money was there. I realized before too long that I was now using six to ten bags a day and, honestly, I was not happy. I wasn't enjoying my life; I was just surviving.

Heroin was a big part of my life, and I had more new people calling me with their 'orders'. So I started buying bricks because I wanted to help people so that they would not be sick. After making sure no one was sick, I would eat a little bit, but I was throwing up a lot.

I was using more and more dope, and at times, panicked because I'd barely had enough for the next day. I was out of control and in a downward spiral. Usually, I was so high that I couldn't even nod off. The highlight of my day was going to my non-dope buddies and smoking a joint with them.

After about three months of this lifestyle, things continued to unravel. My eyes had no sheen in them. My skin was turning yellow. I could barely keep water or food down.

It was getting really 'hot' in the city. More and more busts were being made and my suppliers were becoming unreliable. I tried hard not to get busted and keep my buyers safe. I'd make a few deliveries, mix up the houses, meet in alleys, and at pop machines... but my options were dwindling.

I hated selling drugs. It was a full-time job, and I had nothing to show for it. If I was clean, I could be making money, but I wasn't clean. I wanted out, but I had gotten myself into one hell of a trap. The trap would eventually collapse due to many days without a good supply and because the money was not there. I knew I was in a bad situation. I just had no idea how bad things really were.

Enter the saga of 'sticky fingers'. I have always been creative, but it would work against me in this instance. Now, I was a full-fledged junkie. However, up until this point, I could cover up my habit. Other than stealing my dad's change every now and then or

76

some change from unlocked cars, I didn't cross any of my moral lines. I didn't pressure girls into doing things they normally wouldn't do. I would just give them enough to stay straight and not get sick.

I took care of other people yet, no one was there to help me in my time of need. I had nothing, so I would steal from a few stores when I was sick. Finally, after about a year of stealing to feed my habit, things got so bad my dad had to leave his home because of me. I felt so bad; I just wanted to go to jail.

I never stole from any of my non-junkie friends and tried, even on my worst days of being sick, to have some moral lines. I think down deep I wanted to go to jail because I was getting brave and more reckless and thought I would eventually get caught.

The 'okay days' were spent taking a Suboxone and smoking a few joints with sober friends. Except, more and more, I prayed for death because I just wanted it all to end. I never felt so alone as I did those last weeks. I was waiting for the hammer to fall... for my past to catch up to me. I wondered if it would be a washed check, a fingerprint left behind, or the wrong pawn shop. I already had two shoplifting charges and I was now late on fines. I already needed to do jail time to answer for some of the charges I had against me.

I hit rock bottom, and I hit it hard! I knew I needed to face my self-made fate. I felt like I was dragging on the rocks for a long time. Then one day, my dad called me, and he said, "I can get you into rehab." He asked me if I wanted to go... if I was willing to go. I didn't know that there were rehabs everywhere; all it took was insurance to get into one. I had no idea that this was an option. I tried a Suboxone clinic a few years back and was put on a very long waiting list. So, I told my dad, "Yeah. I want to, and I need the help."

A couple of weeks later and a handful more times of getting 'messed up', I was in a van and on my way to a rehab. On the way there, some guy offered me Clonazepam. He gave me a few, and the next 48 hours were very spotty. I missed the 3-hour bus ride and came to when they did the strip search.

The first two days of my detox, all I did was sleep. Then, as time went on, it went from bad to worse. I had sweats, and chills, and I was sick. It was pretty bad. It was the worst I've ever felt in my life... no joke. During the day, I was feeling okay but things seemed to get worse at night. The sickness, the dreams, the restless legs, the sweats, the chills, the body aches... I tried to keep myself as busy as I could. During the groups, I would listen to the others and, yes, I could relate. I wanted to get clean, but I wanted that one last high.

Things changed though when I was close to finishing rehab. I had a much better attitude and got the tools I needed so that I could use them in the 'real world'. I prayed that my past would not catch up to me.

When I got out of rehab, I stayed with my stoner friend, smoked some herb, and was just happy I was feeling okay. Later, some dope friends came over, but I mustered all of my energy and said no, so they left. I am not sure how this happened to this day, but I had the energy and willpower to say no. I had two jobs and didn't do anything but smoke a little weed. To be honest, it was a fight every day. One that I lost about 40 days after leaving rehab... of course, I blamed it on the pain.

I overdosed pretty badly, and the Narcan was not enough. It took adrenalin to bring me back. It was then that I finally realized I could not save myself without getting help again. I had somewhat broken the physical addiction, but I had a lot going on mentally that I needed to work out. In the back of my mind, I also knew I had 60 days of jail coming up.

I started taking Suboxone every day after the overdose. Just a Suboxone and a couple of joints, and I was doing well. So, with my sentence looming over me, I did what any reasonable person would do. I moved into the woods. With a good friend's help, I lived there for three weeks and felt well.

When I left the woods, I swore to God, who defended me and protected me, that I would live up to a promise and I would never do heroin again. To this day, I have kept that promise. I have not done heroin for 11 years.

I stayed on Suboxone for 4 months after the adventure in the woods and relapsed for a split second. Then I got back into a Suboxone clinic and, for five years, everything has been going well.

I still have herniated discs and many other issues from the car accident. In fact, I'm waiting to get a surgeon who can fix my back. I can honestly say that without Suboxone, my life would have been over. Suboxone made the cravings, pain, and withdrawals all doable. I am healthy, and I live a drug-free lifestyle.

Without Suboxone, I don't think I could have achieved this. My soul is healed. My mind is rewired and, as time goes on, I get stronger and better. Being in nature has allowed me to connect with God. Suboxone has paved the way to being healthy and living my best life possible!

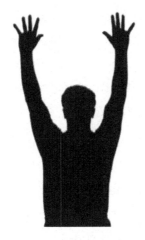

CHAPTER FIVE

The Deep Dark Hole

Anonymous

"Character cannot be developed in ease and quiet. Only through experience of trial and suffering can the soul be strengthened, ambition inspired, and success achieved."

– Helen Keller

This story is a part of my life where I fell into a deep, dark hole. I remember the day just like it was yesterday when I took my first pill. In the summer of '98, I graduated high school, and my mother and father both had knee surgery. Before graduating, someone gave me a Physician's Desk Reference (PDR) and asked me if I had access to certain pills. Of course, I was clueless at the time. I said if I see any, I will let them know.

Time passes and no pills ever show up. Graduation came and went, and I remembered I had the PDR. So, I looked up the medications my parents had in their cupboard, and lo and behold, I found Percocet, which had been there for months and had never been touched. So, one day, I was bored and said screw it. I'm going to take a few. After that day, my life changed forever, not for the better... but for the worse.

The feeling was incredible. It felt as though I was slipping into a hot bath all over my body. It lasted all day, and to be honest, I loved how it felt. I continued to take them until there was no more to take. At the time, I didn't know I would need them just to get through the day. I had no idea how bad the pill 'sickness' would be, and I was in way over my head.

Months went by without any pills, and I wanted to find a way to get some more. Then, one day at work, someone asked me, "Have you ever taken a pill?" and I said, "Hell yeah, what do you got?" He said, "Did you ever hear of Oxycontin?" I had never heard of it, so I asked what it does. The co-worker said it makes you feel as though you're drunk. Who does not like that feeling?!

So, a couple of weeks went by, and then one evening, he asked me if I wanted to do some Oxy 80. I thought, 'why not'. So, he crushed it up, handed me a straw, and I inhaled it through my nose. I was scared at first, but that shit hit me like a ton of bricks. I felt like I was walking on clouds. It made me feel 100 times better than any Percocet that I took previously.

As I am writing this, I am still getting the chill of the effect that the powder feels as it hits the back of my throat. We did some more, off and on, for a few months, and everything was good. I remember getting off the midnight shift, lying in bed, tossing, and turning. So, I took a shower to relax, and get some sleep. It was not happening. I believe that day, my body was telling me that I was having opiate withdrawal symptoms. I ignored the warning signs.

When I went to work, I told my co-worker that I couldn't sleep, and he told me, "You are dope sick." I asked him, "What the hell is that?" He answered, "Your body needs the pill to feel right." At the time, I thought he didn't know what he was talking about. Later, I found out that he was right.

By the summer of 2000, I was a full-blown addict. I was still working but I was always on the hunt for more pills. I had connections to a few guys from work who had access to a 'flow line' of pills. So, I went for months getting Oxy, Percocet, and a drug called 'rockets'. Then they introduced me to more people, and the supply never ended.

Eventually, everyone in town knew the doctors who ran the 'pill mills'. I jumped on board and scheduled my first doctor's appointment. I still remember being scared because I thought he wouldn't give me anything. Boy, I was wrong! This dude gave me enough pills to knock out horses. I felt like I hit the jackpot. In just one visit, I got 60 Oxy 80's, and 300 Roxy 30's.

At first, that lasted a little more than a month. Three months had passed, and I started taking more and more… ultimately, always ending up empty towards the end of the month.

At this point, the craving and withdrawals were full-blown. I couldn't sleep. I couldn't function. I had sweats and chills. I was irritable, agitated, and sore everywhere. I was a full-blown addict with a wife and two young boys. The struggles ahead of me are not yet seen but will be shortly.

I went to this doctor for seven years. Then, in January 2006, I went to get my script, and his office was closed. I later found out that he was on the run from over-scripting. My life went on a downhill spiral.

Within three months, I lost my job, my house, and my car, all from not paying the bills and using the money to buy pills. I stayed in the home until the Sherriff came and kicked me out. My wife and boys moved in with her parents. I would visit when I could, but these were very deep and dark times. I couldn't get any pills on my own. So, I was constantly scheming everyone out of everything.

Until late 2007, I lived on and off the streets until my parents let me move in with them. They said I could stay if I was working. They didn't know about my addiction. And I'm now living with my brother and sister, who are also addicts. Now I have two people who have contacts, and we can share our resources.

Life was kind of on track until April 21, 2008. This day almost took me off this earth, but God had a different plan for me. That morning I was going to work and was involved in a head-on collision that came very close to killing me. I don't remember anything except thinking I was in a dream with music playing. When I thought I was merely waking up, I was really coming out of a coma.

It was a big shock!

I got really jacked up from the accident, but the drugs were plentiful, so it was an addict's paradise. I was on so many painkillers I didn't know what day it was.

As time passed, my family would come to visit. My siblings were nodding off, and I knew something wasn't right.

When I came home a few months later, I discovered that my brother and sister were shooting dope. So now I am back home with a shitload of meds, and I am using them all day, every day... once again.

My regular doctor prescribed the meds, but he told me I would have to see pain management to fill them. He recommended a pain management doctor, and I was good to go! I rode that wave a couple of years, then I was called in for a pill count. I went there without any pills, so they discharged me from their services the same day. So here we go again... no pills...

I was fed up with feeling terrible, sick, having no money... having nothing. I struggled every day on all fronts. So, one day, in 2012, I walked through the doors of a local Methadone clinic here in my hometown. That day, my life changed forever... and all for the better.

Many people said to me that I was exchanging one drug for another. At first, I thought that they were right. But, in time, I found that if you work the program the way it's designed, want to be clean, get the counseling and follow their recommendations, the program works miracles. I am living proof!

My sister died from a drug overdose, and my brother was in prison for over 5 years. I asked myself why my sister was gone and why it wasn't me? There were plenty of times I should have overdosed, but I pulled through. Today, as I write this, I know she is watching over me and proud of how I live. She is happy that I am drug-free and that I got my life back. This is truly the best I have felt in years. Yes, it may have taken me years to finish my treatment, but I did it, and I have never looked back.

If a person wants help, they can get it. The treatment and counseling I received gave me the tools to improve and get better. I could be dead or in jail which are the alternatives to the drug lifestyle, but I thank God for how this unfolded. To you, the reader, that may be struggling...

There is hope!

People who give clinics a bad rap don't have a clue. They lack education, information, and knowledge. Please don't think bad of me. Most people are very proud of me. I'm very proud of myself. There are judgmental people wherever you go that impact our perception of things. You never hear about the people who excel, do well, and turn their lives around because they are the quiet ones that just try to do all they can to have a productive, drug-free lifestyle.

I have been out of the clinic for a few years now and I know not to let my guard down... ever. I am drug-free, clean, and responsible. I like the person I am today. My life has fallen back together as it should be. I am also aware that if I need help again, God forbid, I have resources here in my small hometown and will never be judged. I can get help if needed from very dedicated people who care. I hope, by reading this, you get a different outlook on the Methadone clinic or any other clinics available to help people with addictions.

Thanks to these services, understand that lives are being saved every single day, including mine!

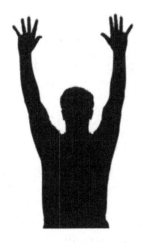

CHAPTER SIX

Yours For the Taking

By Jenn

"Though no one can go back and make a brand-new start, anyone can start from now and make a brand-new ending."

– Carl Bard

My mother was fifteen when she found out she was pregnant and had me when she turned sixteen. Her dad was a raging alcoholic, and he worked a shitty shift work job at the paper mill. He was always yelling, getting drunk, and abusing my grandmother and their three daughters.

When my grandmother was nine years old, she was afflicted with polio, affecting her legs. She suffered most of her life. My mom did what she could do for us, but she still went out with her friends since she was still a teenager.

My dad and mom were married when my mother was eight months pregnant with me. They were divorced when I was three. My dad lived with his parents, about an hour and a half from my mother and me.

I went back and forth between the grandparents' homes most of my childhood. I never understood why my mother would leave me with my mean alcoholic grandfather so much, but maybe she didn't have a choice. Although he was never mean to me, my grandfather was scary. Years later, I found out that my grandfather had been sexually molested by his father. Unfortunately, many neighborhood kids had been molested by him too.

Eventually, my great-grandfather was sent to a mental institution for two years, where he received electric shock therapy. However, after he returned home, the same molesting behavior continued. So, my grandfather left home.

My mother and I struggled just to keep food on the table. I remember sitting on the floor in the bathroom eating and coloring because we could only afford to heat that tiny space. Our apartment was full of spiders and other bugs. My mother had a heated waterbed, so we spent a lot of time there. This was my first experience with what I called 'the jerks'. Now I know it is sleep paralysis.

I was five years old and recall being awake in my head, but my body was asleep. I couldn't move or talk and was terrified. I told my mom what I felt, and she just looked at me funny. It continues to this day, but not as intense as when I was young.

My parents were sharing custody of me, but I spent most of my time with both sets of grandparents. Then, when I was six, my dad and his parents moved to south Florida, and my mother met a man, Tom, from Kentucky. My mother married him when I was eight. A few months later, my mother had a baby girl.

Things were going great in Kentucky. We had enough food, never cold, and I had my own room. Dreams do come true!

My dad was working odd jobs in a couple of hotels in south Florida. This is where he became very acquainted with the South Florida drug trade. He knew there was a lot of money, and he wanted some of it for himself.

I would visit him during the summer breaks. Luckily, my father was still living with his parents, so I was protected. However, his parents eventually moved, and my father was left to his own devices and his newfound trade. During my summer vacations there, I began frequenting the bars and attending parties with my now drug-trading father.

My father had so much money. We would ride in limousines, eat filet mignon, and shop like crazy. But the opposite was also true. We lived in an efficiency apartment, walked everywhere, and ate bread and mayo sandwiches. I finally asked him what he did for a living, and he told me the truth. In fact, he told me too much.

As a teenager, I thought it was 'cool' that my father did what he did. I had no rules, could do whatever I wanted, whenever I wanted, and had no chores. At the time, it was a teenager's dream come true.

When returning home to Kentucky, the scenario was much different. My stepfather and mother had rules, curfew, chores, and church activities. It was totally different than living with my dad because my stepfather, who I began to call dad, did what was right.

My biological dad suffered from anxiety and depression and was an addict. The last summer I spent with him he was called to go on a trip to Columbia. I was supposed to wait for him to return home. But instead, I decided to go home to Kentucky. He never answered his phone, so I didn't call to let him know I had left.

One of his friends tried to contact him, and he wasn't answering his phone. So, he went around to the back of his apartment. He looked in his bedroom window to find my dad lying on the floor. His friend heard my dad's last words, "I think I am dying." And he did.

When my mother and I went to the house to clean it out, many things were missing. I am pretty sure the Columbian cartel got into the house to get rid of the things they needed... the guns, drugs, scales, and his wallet. People from the cartel were trying to contact me. On the back door, there was a note. It read, "Duane, we will know we've been crossed if we don't hear from you in 24 hours." The police called me twice, wanting to know what I knew about my father's activities. I never called them back.

Upon his passing, I discovered that the boat used to transport drugs was in my name! The Columbians were calling me non-stop, wanting to fly a friend and me to Miami, so I could sign the 42-foot Hatteras over to them. It was a terrifying time. I did not know who to trust! Besides, there's no way my mom and stepfather would send me back to Florida.

As I got older and began having my own kids, I began to feel angry toward my biological father. I would never have my kids in a bar at age 13. The lifestyle that I had with my father impacted my life. However, I promised myself that I would not be a prisoner of my past. That it was a lesson, not a life sentence. When I look back at my father's mistakes, I try to learn from them.

I had a rocky relationship with my stepdad, who I consider my real dad. Since getting clean three years ago, I've been able to genuinely appreciate what he tried to do. We now have a great relationship, and I feel truly blessed to have him in my life. I am thankful he has stuck with me my entire life, even after he and my mother divorced. He never changed and is still supportive to this day!

I am a mother to two boys; one is seven, and the other is nineteen. I am a sister, a friend, and an animal lover. I love to read, go to the beach, kayak, and the movies. Unfortunately, I am also an addict. I believe I am a good person but haven't always made the best choices when dealing with my addiction. Thankfully my family has forgiven me for lying, stealing, and not coming home for weeks at a time.

The hardest part for me is forgiving myself. I've been clean from pain pills (opioids) for three years, four months, and five days. I care about myself again. When you look your best, you feel good about yourself again.

When I was in full addiction, I only cared about whatever drug I needed to feel better. How was I going to get money and find the drugs? What was I going to do with my son while looking for drugs? I look back at it today and honestly can't believe I made it out alive!!

Here is how my addiction started…

I was diagnosed with depression and anxiety when I was nineteen years old. Although I had felt depressed most of my life, I noticed it even more when my biological father passed away. I was placed on anti-depressants, seeing a therapist, and things were looking up. I was working, had a lovely apartment, my own car, credit cards, and was close to my family. I was drinking some and smoking pot, but nothing I thought was crazy.

After about three years, the medication for my depression stopped working. I tried about 20 different drugs and saw a lot of different doctors, and nothing seemed to help me. I basically fell into bed for the next ten years or maybe longer. My husband took care of our four-year-old son and me. I hated myself at this point, so I didn't take a shower, brush my teeth, brush my hair, or leave my house. My family would call, and I would just hang up on them. I felt like a piece of shit just rotting away. I didn't want to kill myself, but I knew I didn't want to keep living how I was living.

Depression, anxiety, and mental illness took hold of me and held me hostage. It was torture in my own head. Finally, I thought of cutting myself just to feel something different. I did try, but it just didn't work the way I thought it would.

My husband found a different doctor who prescribed Effexor, Adderall, and Xanax for me. The Adderall, taken in the morning and afternoon, got me out of bed and made me feel on top of the world. However, I had no idea Adderall was like meth! It keeps you up, and I liked it!! Pretty soon, I was taking more than what I was prescribed. I loved the feeling of being out of bed and doing things.

Then it began to hurt my life. I made terrible choices, staying up for days, and I lost sixty pounds. I was 102 pounds and stood at five feet nine inches. I looked skeletal. I started going to bars and hanging out all night. I loved the feeling of the Adderall, so I wasn't using the Xanax at all. I enjoyed the Adderall too much. I felt like I was finally out of bed and living!

I was not living the good, honest life I dreamed about. I wasn't taking care of my son, now nine or ten. I didn't come home for a week, nor did I call my family. I began cheating on the man who loved me, cared for me, and cared for our son. I was out of control and only thinking of myself. I continued running around all night selling my Xanax to buy more Adderall off the street. I was having the time of my life! I was drinking, hanging out with people I thought were my friends, and not taking care of myself, my son, or my family.

After about two years, my family called my doctor and told her I was abusing my medication. As a result, I was taken off all meds and went to my first rehab facility in Atlanta, Georgia.

After treatment, I returned home and fell in bed with my depression and anxiety. I started going to an outpatient program. It helped me get out of the house and be around people who understood what I was going through.

I was placed on different anti-depressants, but nothing seemed to help. I stopped going to meetings and stayed in bed. My husband would bring me food, and my son would come to sit with me. It was beyond sad. My husband took my son to school, went to work, took care of the house and all the chores, and took him to his activities; t-ball, boy scouts, baseball, everything!! He was raising my son by himself. I missed all my son's activities and couldn't do anything for anyone or myself.

My family tried to be supportive, but they were all in different states and didn't know precisely how to help me. At this point, many of my family members were just glad they knew where I was and that I wasn't out partying. I missed the Adderall feeling but knew that wasn't the way. Besides, it wasn't a choice any longer.

On my way to see a new psychiatrist, I was rear-ended by another car. My head hit the steering wheel very hard, and I was taken to the hospital by ambulance. I had damage to the cervical 2nd, 3rd, & 4th vertebrae. I was given some Vicodin and the name of a doctor and chiropractor to see. At my first doctor's appointment, I was prescribed 90-30 mg of Oxycontin, which I was to take three times a day. This started another struggle with pain pills. Like the Adderall, I felt great and on top of the world. I could get out of bed, do things, go places, and take care of my son. I was in love with the feeling!!

Once again, I started taking more than the specified amount and, eventually, started snorting them. Soon, I was on the streets looking for more to buy.

Again, I felt great and began partying with my so-called 'friends'. Unfortunately, I wasn't coming home or calling home either. Going through the hell of withdrawals, I started lying, cheating, and stealing from the people I loved. I never thought I would sink this low, but I did.

My husband wanted full custody of my son, which was the best decision, but I fought it. So, I moved in with a girlfriend for a few months, putting my son in danger. Eventually, my family stepped in, and we tried to come up with a plan. Then, I found out I was pregnant. Initially, I wasn't happy about it. I was 42 years old, doing drugs, and not living a healthy lifestyle.

When I was 3 months pregnant, I had to quit cold turkey. I didn't think I could do it, but it wasn't only about me anymore. I moved back in with my husband and son. The withdrawals were terrible. I'm used to lying in bed, so that's what I did until I gave birth in January. By the grace of God, my second son was born healthy.

The first year with my son was easy. I struggled with depression and insomnia, but a baby just needs to be breastfed, held, and have his diaper changed. As he developed and began crawling, I struggled to take care of him. I was just so exhausted, so tired, I could barely take care of myself, let alone a child.

Once again, I tried some different anti-depressants. Unfortunately, my insomnia was also getting out of control, so I was committed to the hospital for help. I needed help but was having difficulty reaching out for it, and the hospital experience did not help. I just couldn't do it. I was in my head way too much, and it was getting scarier and scarier by the minute.

People, family, and loved ones can't read your mind, but I still felt they should have known how I felt. They should have done something. I now know you must speak up. Let people know what you need, and there are people out there to help.

At this point, no one knew I was on Suboxone. However, everyone knew about my past with addiction, depression, and anxiety. I still felt judged by everyone, but looking back now, I realize I was the one judging them, and I was judging myself.

One day my sister and I were driving to her doctor's appointment, and we started talking about my struggles. I told her I wasn't happy with myself and didn't want to live with this pain anymore. Pain, meaning my depression and anxiety. She asked if I had a plan to kill myself. I told her that I did. I had thought of two ways I would do it. The reality was that I didn't want to die, but I just didn't want to live how I was living. I was doing my best and wasn't happy with it. Now, death scares the living shit out of me!

Immediately, my sister talked to the rest of the family. They knew I needed some serious help. It was decided I would move to Seattle with my youngest sister for a while until we could find a place for me to get help with my depression, anxiety, and my life. I needed to take better care of myself all the way around, including diet and exercise.

While being with my sister for three months, I started going to Alcoholics Anonymous/Narcotics Anonymous (AA/NA) meetings weekly. I went to yoga classes, support groups, smart recovery meetings, and more AA/NA meetings. On the weekends, I would spend time with my son going for walks, to the parks, and on adventures.

My family found a place that dealt with everything I needed help with called The Center, A Place of Hope. My husband took my son home with him, and I went to The Center. I lived in a nice house with five girls. We got up at 8 A.M., went to many classes, and learned about Cognitive Behavior Therapy and Developmental Behavior Therapy. Both therapies have been very valuable, and I still use them today. I stayed at the center for 6 weeks and was still on the Suboxone when I returned home.

I was down to one strip a day but eventually fell back into bed and started selling my Suboxone for money to get Oxycontin. This went on for almost a year before I couldn't take it any longer. Finally, I called a local treatment center, The Discovery House, to get the help I needed. I was given Methadone, and I felt like a new person. I ended up on 23mg of Methadone a day, which was over 3 years ago.

As I write this now, I have a job, two friends I love and trust, and, most importantly, I am happy where I am. I genuinely like myself!

My family and I have never been in a better place. If I become sad or depressed, I use the tools I've learned over the years. Every day isn't perfect, but it's perfect to me!! Years ago when I was 'doing my best,' I hated my best. When I'm doing my best now, I am happy with my best!! I give my best to myself, my boys, and my family every day.

If you're struggling in the throes of addiction, depression, or anxiety, don't think that you are alone. Instead, reach out to a doctor or a friend. Find a program because plenty are ready and willing to support you. Do your research until you find the one that works for you.

What are your dreams and goals? What do you want for your life, the life you've been given? Go out and try different things! Never stop trying! It's been 25 years, and I finally found what works for my family and me.

You can accomplish your dreams, achieve your goals, and do whatever you are passionate about. Looking back at the things you wish you never did is of no use. That is all in the past and can't be changed.

Instead, look forward to your future. It's yours for the taking. It's whatever you choose to make it.

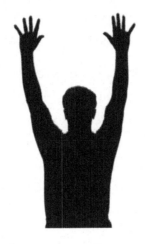

CHAPTER SEVEN

The Rise After the Fall

By Amanda

"Strength does not come from physical capacity. It comes from an indomitable will."

– Mahatma Gandhi

My name is Amanda, and I was born in September 1978. I am 42 years old. I had two older brothers and two younger brothers. Unfortunately, my youngest brother passed away. I also have one older sister who supported me when no one else would. I am incredibly thankful for her.

When I was seven, my eldest brother started to molest me. This abuse went on until I was ten. I was frozen and couldn't tell a single soul. I repressed it until much later in life. However, I don't believe that's why I became an addict. So many people have experienced trauma and didn't turn to drugs and alcohol. Currently, I am in a rehab facility in Pennsylvania.

I grew up living in a trailer with my siblings. We didn't have structure or discipline growing up. I got picked on at home and at school. The clothes I wore were hand-me-downs, and some were from thrift stores. I didn't have what everyone else had and never felt like I fit in. I always wanted to be someone else, and I fantasized about it often. I always asked God why I had the parents I had and why they couldn't be different.

In fifth grade, a boy had a crush on me and wow, did I love the attention! The problem was I didn't like him. I didn't have the heart to tell him because I didn't want to hurt his feelings and loved the attention. To this day, I struggle with putting myself first. I am a people pleaser.

When I was thirteen, I took my first drink of alcohol, and I loved it. My anxiety disappeared, and I felt confident like I could take on the world. The morning after drinking, I always said I would never do it again, but I did. Within two weeks, I was smoking marijuana and drinking. At fifteen, I had a back injury and was prescribed pain medication. After having back surgery, I could get any narcotic I wanted and didn't realize the dangers of getting addicted.

At sixteen, I started snorting cocaine. I was drinking and doing cocaine with a few friends in a hotel room. The next thing I knew, I was waking up in a hospital with my mother sitting beside me. I died three times in the ambulance from alcohol poisoning.

During my entire teenage years and some of my adult life, I replaced love with sex. I don't think I knew what love was until I was in my mid-thirties.

When I was seventeen, I was introduced to crack cocaine, and I thought I found the love of my life. However, it almost took my life multiple times. I've been getting high on and off for twenty-five years. I have had some clean times here and there, six years one time, four years another, only to relapse. This is my twentieth time in rehab. I have stayed clean for twenty-eight days on two different occasions. Usually, I was able to manipulate my way out of rehab. Currently, I have been in rehab for sixty–eight days. At this point, I am living day by day.

I am taking recovery advice from everyone. Some people have been clean for one day, and others have been clean for ten years. It really doesn't matter how long they've been clean. You can be clean for twenty-five years but your just as close to relapse as the person who's been clean one day. It doesn't matter where you hear the message, because that message may keep you clean for that day. You have to be open-minded enough to understand and believe the message you receive.

I want to go back and fill in a few missing pieces. When I was fourteen, I was at a friend's house, and his parents were out of town. There was a lot of alcohol, pot, and pills. Before the night was over, I passed out on the parent's bed. I'm not sure how I got there, but I assume someone carried me. When I woke up, someone was having sex with me... or better said, raping me. I didn't not consent to this and for years, I didn't know it was rape. I thought it was my fault because I was drunk. I thought maybe I said yes, but I was too intoxicated to make that choice even if I did. I was fourteen years old, and he was over eighteen. I've carried this my whole life until now. I finally shared this abuse with my counselor and my peers. The weight has been lifted off my shoulders.

In November of 2020, I was raped again, but this time was able to deal with it more effectively. Although, I haven't pressed charges yet. That is my next step and the only way I will be able to get closure.

I wanted to share these things because no matter what you have been through there is always someone who has been through worse. Even from my situation, I have heard stories far more dramatic than mine, and they have gotten through it. It's not easy, but it's worth it.

I have a seventeen-year-old son and six-year-old daughter, and they are amazing kids! My son hates drugs because he saw what it did to me. And now I'm doing what it takes so my daughter will never see me high.

The disease of addiction has defeated me. It took everything from me. Before I came here, I was homeless in a neighborhood I had no business being in. All the things I said I'd never do, I did. All my 'nevers' happened, so yes, I'm defeated. I'm desperate, and the pain is unbearable, so I'm ready to change my life.

They say, "When the pain is great enough, you'll change" or "When the pain of staying the same is greater than the pain of change, you'll change."

I couldn't live one more day the way I was living. What addiction has done to me is beyond what I can comprehend. Towards the end of my addiction, I would take anything you gave me to numb me. I didn't care if I knew what it was or not. I'd sleep with anyone to get money or drugs, even if I didn't know them. It is only by the grace of God I don't have any sexually-transmitted diseases and I am still alive.

I've overdosed on heroin nine times. But God has a purpose for me!

I'm finally ready and willing to put all my energy into recovery, no matter what the cost. The rewards of staying clean are priceless! Finally, I can look in the mirror and like who is looking back at me.

If you are struggling, there are twenty-four-hour hotlines you can call. Some are listed in this book for your reference. If you're struggling, make the call. You are worth it!!

For me, the pain of using was greater than the pain of changing. That's when I knew I was ready. The disease won, destroyed me, and broke me down. But, on the other side of this is the rise after the fall.

I am a completely different, better, version of myself. I am getting my own place and my daughter is coming to live with me. I have a great support group here and a new attitude. I will continue with the Alcoholics Anonymous/Narcotics Anonymous program so I can continue to heal. Don't ever be ashamed to ask for help. It won't be easy, but it will be worth it!

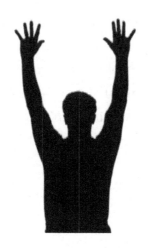

CHAPTER EIGHT

Little by Little… One Day at a Time

By Anonymous

"Nothing is impossible; the word itself says, 'I'm possible!'"

– Audrey Hepburn

I've been clean from heroin since March 21, 2017. When I was getting high, the only thing that mattered was dope. I didn't care what happened to me. I didn't care if I died. As long as I died high, I'd be happy. I put myself in situations I never imagined and hurt so many people in the process. As a kid you have dreams. You think about what you want to be when you grow up. You don't think you'll become an addict. You don't expect drugs to take over your entire life.

Growing up, my childhood wasn't the greatest. I come from a broken home. My sister helped raise me. My mom and dad didn't have the best relationship. My dad had a really hard time staying faithful. One time, I showed my mom my dad's friend's house, not knowing it was one of his girlfriend's houses. My dad eventually left. I think he felt bad. He tried to buy my love instead of spending time with me. My mom worked a lot and did her best, given what life threw her way. However, I often felt like the problem child. I didn't feel seen or heard.

During my freshman year of high school, my dad got really sick and passed away from Cirrhosis of the liver. Around the same time, when I was playing soccer, I ended up tearing my anterior cruciate and medial collateral ligaments. The doctor prescribed Percocet and right away I knew I loved the feeling it gave me. Eventually, I started smoking weed and drinking. Life seemed better that way. After my dad died, I found out he had his own struggles with drugs.

When I was 17, I started partying and taking pills. I was tired of school, but I did graduate. For the longest time, I was hooked on having something up my nose… then came the needle.

Getting drugs was easy back then because my boyfriend always knew where to get it. That toxic relationship ended 3 years later. In fact, every relationship I had was toxic. I experienced emotional and physical abuse. To this day I am still struggling to heal from what I experienced.

I went to a private college for a while but got kicked out. My addiction came first. So, I worked as a waitress, and I bartended here and there. My tips were usually used to get pills and dope. I thought I was doing good at the time. Even though I had a job, the money I was making wasn't enough to support my habit. So, I started stealing from my employer, family, and the guys who

105

liked me. Then, I got involved with a guy I worked with, and I introduced him to dope. That toxic relationship lasted for 3 years or so.

My addiction was pretty bad at that point. We were both a mess And I ended up getting pregnant. When I told him, he was so happy, and I was crying. He thought a baby was the answer to all of our problems. Lying, stealing from people, boosting, pawning... sometimes not knowing where to stay or go. He was telling me we could handle it and that I should be excited. I wasn't. In fact, I was terrified about bringing a baby into the picture.

I was three months pregnant and decided I didn't want a baby, so I ended the pregnancy. I went into a McDonalds bathroom immediately afterward and got high. This was a choice I never thought I'd make. A choice I never want to be faced with ever again. Don't get me wrong. I always wanted to be a mom. However, at that time, dying high seemed like the better choice.

I finally decided to go to rehab. I didn't like the way I was living anymore. My boyfriend kept using. I thought I could handle it when I got back home. Finally, after 30 days in rehab, I was ready to handle life sober. Yet, a day after I got home, I ended up calling him. I relapsed, getting high once again.

Since I got back from rehab, my mom was on my case. I wasn't working so I decided to leave and move in with him. I was still doing drugs, so I had to find ways to get the money to buy them. I did what I did best. I lied, boosted, and stole from people again.

I would drive back and forth to Detroit, staying in run down places or motels. I watched my boyfriend, and other people overdose right in front of me. A friend I was with the night before was found dead the next morning. People close to me were losing their lives to drugs.

I was out of rehab for a few months, and my boyfriend wanted me to go back. He told me this time he'd do it with me. We'd get clean together and learn to be the people we wanted to be. Honestly, I didn't want to go back, but he begged me. The way we were living, we knew one of us, or both of us, would end up dead.

Reluctantly, I checked into rehab again and we planned on getting sober. We planned on moving so we could get a fresh start. Just a few days before I was discharged, he called me from another rehab facility and told me he couldn't be with me anymore. He wanted me to have a chance to be happy and was afraid that we wouldn't be good for each other. I didn't know how to process all of that. My counselor suggested I stay for another 45 days. I figured I didn't have anything to lose, so I stayed. Later, I found out I had Hepatitis C.

When my 45 days were up, I went back home and got into an intensive outpatient program. I went five days a week. Eventually, I got on a maintenance program, and have been living life one day at a time ever since. I try not to get ahead of myself. I try not to live in the past. I make sure that I don't make the same choices I did when I was addicted. Today, I am a totally different person. I continue to work on healing and becoming all that I can be... little by little, one day at a time.

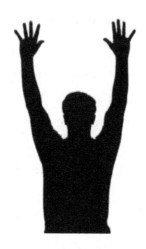

CHAPTER NINE

Prayers Do Get Answered

By Steve

"The only person you are destined to become is the person you decide to be."

– Ralph Waldo Emerson

Hello, my name is Steve. I grew up in a dysfunctional family with an alcoholic father and a mother who struggled to raise three boys. Initially, I attended St. Mary's Catholic School. I went to church every Sunday and was an altar boy. As a kid, I was always seeking attention because, at the time, my father was never around. He was either at the bar or drinking at home. At home, we were always on the end of his 'bad days.' I remember he would take us to the basement and beat us with a two-by-four for being loud or just being kids. I was terrified of him! I remember when he would fight with my mother, I would run into the woods and cry. I'd stay there until it was dark, then I'd return home.

When we switched schools, I struggled because I didn't fit in. Aside from wearing hand-me-downs, I struggled in school and was not a good communicator. I tried sports, but that didn't turn out well, so I joined the chorus. There was a girl in chorus I liked. We used to take field trips to sing to old people and it was an easy way out of class.

My father's side of the family drank a lot. By age eleven, I was stealing my parent's cigarettes and sneaking drinks at family parties. The first time I got drunk I made wine spritzers for my aunt. I would sip the wine as I was making them. That night, I got very sick and threw up. I can still remember laying on the car floor all the way home. Once home, I continued to throw up. Despite this, I would sneak out at night and try to steal my dad's beer. I would check the beer bottles he left on the coffee table to see if any beer was left. I thought I had gotten lucky once and found a full bottle of beer. I started to drink it really fast so I wouldn't get caught. To my dismay, the bottle was full of cigarette butts. Once again, I was running to the bathroom to throw up. Still, that didn't stop me from trying to get that next drink. I would steal drinks at parties, look for drinks people didn't finish and steal beer from my father.

My mother became friends with my neighbor's brother, who also drank a lot. We would go out to Moraine State Park with him. There I would sit on the hood of his car and drink Mezcal. At that time, I thought this was the coolest thing in the world. This went on for a while and I enjoyed every minute of it.

One of my brothers moved out of the house and into my uncle's house, so I started to hang out with my other older brother, Ryan and his friend. My mother made him take me with him. I think she was trying to keep me away from my drunk father. My brother and his friend smoked a lot of weed. I started smoking it too, and I loved it.

When I was in ninth grade, I started to take Klonipin. In school, I would either swallow them or snort them. Sometimes, I'd get home from school and pass out for two days. I probably overdosed but my mom was working so much she didn't notice.

My parents were fighting a lot then too. My father would slam my mother into walls. After one particular fight, we waited until my father went to work then we packed up everything in the house. We left him with one chair. It was very difficult to deal with all the craziness at the time. So, I started going downhill with the pills. I didn't fit in and was getting into more and more trouble in school. Aside from having a fucked-up family, it was embarrassing, and I was ashamed that I didn't have a family like some of my friends.

I smoked dope in the school bathrooms and wood shop and started taking more pills. Of course, getting in trouble in school goes without saying. I would pretend that I was going to school. But as soon as my mom left for work, I would go back home, drink, sleep, or just hang out. I was actively looking for people to buy beer from so I could party all day. By tenth grade, I was failing my classes. My mom caught on, and I had to go to summer school. Even so, I still managed to party most of the day. I was out of control, but I thought I had it licked. But I was in a dark place. Yeah, I was the cool kid, skipping school and partying all night...

110

what a joke. What I didn't understand was that I was ruining my life.

The fights with my mother became more frequent because she was tired of the partying and all the dumb shit going on. Well, I met a girl who appeared to be financially well off. Her mom was a cocaine dealer, and I started to live with her and her mom. They had a lot of money, and I got what I wanted, cars, trucks and, of course, drugs. I dropped out of school in the eleventh grade and kept partying until I discovered my girlfriend was sleeping with my friends. So, I broke up with her and moved back to my mother's house. I enrolled back in school and took some extra classes. I managed to graduate with all A's and B's!

My mother and I continued to fight over my partying, and I was just too much for her to handle. It didn't really matter to me, so I kept partying. I did manage to get a maintenance job at Butler Community College. My father wouldn't give me a ride, so I walked for 45 minutes to and from work every day. Eventually, I received an offer to attend University Technical Institute for Auto Mechanics. My mother was thrilled and took me to visit the school. My mother helped with the school loan, and my father helped me buy a truck.

While at school, I got a job in construction. At the same time, I met some people who were selling cocaine. So, I started selling cocaine on the job as well as using my own supply. Unfortunately, I was running out of money because I was using more than I was selling. I got fired for stealing, ended up quitting school and moved back to my mother's house. Luckily, the landlord let me do work for him around the apartment building.

One day I was hanging out with my friends at Walmart and saw a car full of girls. I left a note on the car, and the girl driving called me. We had a relationship that didn't end well. I wrecked her car, and we eventually broke up. She was nineteen at the time, and I was twenty. I received a call about eight months later from Bethany Christian Services, an adoption agency. I called the girl's mother to find out what was going on and she started yelling at me. Apparently, she was pregnant, but she never told me. Come to find out, she hid it from everyone, and her mom's boyfriend found her in labor. So, I had to go to the agency to meet with the case worker and sign adoption papers.

When I held my daughter for the first time, I broke down and started to cry. I couldn't understand why my daughter was being taken from me. I signed the adoption papers because I didn't want to fight with her mother for custody.

Storming out of the building, I began driving recklessly, hoping to die in a car wreck. My mom saw me and pulled up beside me. She talked me into pulling over until I calmed down.

After that, I received my second DUI, got into a fight, and got fired from one job after another. I met a new girl and soon after I moved in with her. I worked with her brother, and he drove me to work every day. He was a heavy drinker too so I got drunk with him all the time. So, my girlfriend and I ended up breaking up. I had to move out, but I continued to work with her brother. Eventually, I was on house arrest because I broke into a building. At that time, I met a dude at work who was selling morphine pills. Every payday, I would buy 50 to 100 of them. I was lost when he quit and had to find something else to replace the pills. So, I started taking heroin.

This really took a toll on me. I got fired from my job, cut my foot in half, had fevers, and was doing cocaine and alcohol. Once again, I was kicked out of my living space and moved back in with my mom. My mom bought a new house and one of the neighbors was a druggie. My heroin habit was horrible at the time. I went to the bar with my neighbor and was going through withdrawals. I was so sick that I had him drive me to the dealer's house. I lied to the dealer and told him the money was in the car. I watched him load his gun. When he turned away, I stole the dope, ran to the car, and we sped away. The dealer fired three shots at us, and one landed in the back bumper. Later that night, the dealer smashed the car windows and flattened all the tires.

I met another girl who lived close to my mother, and we started dating. For a minute, I cleaned up my act. However, we fought constantly, so we broke up, and I started using heroin again.

I had an ankle bracelet, was on probation, and working for my neighbor. I stole his guns, failed a urine test, and had to go to rehab. When I got out, I couldn't do heroin because I got the Vivitrol shot, so I started smoking crack.

Eventually, my Vivitrol shot wore off, and I had a bad overdose at my neighbor's house. I woke up to cops and paramedics in my face. Because we live in a small community, my mother already found out that I had overdosed.

The following Monday, I turned myself into my probation officer. At the time, my neighbor realized I stole his guns, and he filed a police report. I spent two years in state prison. While I was there,

I participated in every program they had to offer - Alcoholics Anonymous, Narcotics Anonymous, and church meetings. Generally speaking, I was doing well.

When I got out of prison, I moved back in with the same girl, got my driver's license, a new job, and a truck, and it seemed like I was doing well. I started going to a recovery program, cycling through the steps, and everything was going great. However, I had a lot of unresolved resentment, so the story continues.

I met a man at work who sold cocaine. Coincidentally, I hurt my back, started smoking crack and went off the deep end. Once again, I got fired for stealing and I lied to my girlfriend about it. I found a new job but was still smoking crack. The drug use caught up with me again. I ended up nodding off, wrecking my truck, and getting my fourth DUI. My girlfriend broke up with me that night. Nothing stopped me from using now. I had nothing to lose.

I got another job and was using my mother's truck. I used it to get some dope, but I nodded off again... wrecking her truck by hitting a telephone pole and a tree. I broke my pelvis and had to have surgery. Two weeks later, I was out getting high again. I moved out of my mother's house and began using meth. I pretty much gave up on life at that point.

I had two more overdoses and moved back into my mother's house. I didn't quit using, and I would leave for a week at a time. I would stay with a friend in Butler and sell dope. I sold a bag to a girl who overdosed in the truck outside the house. One of the neighbors called the cops and they took me to jail on an old warrant. I spent two weeks there. My mom bailed me out and I stayed clean for about fifteen days. Then started getting dope again.

One morning, I woke up early to my mom sitting on my bed crying. She thought I was dead because I wasn't answering my phone. This bothered me, so I checked into rehab. As I write this, I have been clean for thirty days. I will keep sharing my story and get the help I need to connect to my higher power. I am going to get a sponsor and work the program. I will do the work I need to do so I can start working in the drug and alcohol field. I want to help other addicts because I feel that it is my purpose.

I will continue praying for addicts in hopes that they get the help they need. And I want to thank everyone who prays, too, because we need your prayers. They do get answered.

This is my story... Steve

CONCLUSION

"The one thing you've gotta do is that you need to always do the best you can do, no matter what the given situation, no matter what comes up against you. You do the best you can do, and you never give up. Never quit."

– James Corden

After many rebounds and relapses, the authors of this book share their stories of getting *'Unhooked'* from the strangle hold of addiction. Many of these authors are doing wonderful! In fact, they are living their best life ever! Unfortunately, one could not overcome the grip of addiction and lost his life. One author is currently fighting a hard battle and her struggles continue.

As they say, we must learn to take a sad song and make it better. We have heard this in the past as a musical lyric, but what does it really mean?! We have all faced our fair share of challenges and difficult times. We often get lost and wonder what to do.

We all have a choice. We can wallow in self-pity and the 'poor me' energy or we can get up and decide to change. It could always be worse!

We must use our challenges to grow and learn from them. No one "has it made" or has the "perfect life". It's about striving to find happiness in everything we can. We must make the right choices to take the necessary steps, even if they're baby steps, to improve our lives. Everyone is responsible for their own happiness, and if you are not happy and want things to change, you must look in the mirror. All of us have met negative people that, without change, will be negative their entire existence. Yes, true, some people can handle things better than others.

The authors in this book share their stories with you to show you what's possible. That change is possible if you're willing to do the work. Is it easy to change? Of course not! But with drive, determination and support, change can and will happen! You simply have to be open-minded to get the help that you need. With support, you can develop the skills you need to overcome major obstacles in your life. If you are willing to change, and you have the desire to, change can happen no matter how helpless and hopeless you feel. It may not happen overnight... it might happen in a matter of days, or it could take months, years or a lifetime.

Life is unfair and challenging, but we must take what we have and do what we need to do to reshape our lives, so the past does not consume our future. We need to learn to process and eliminate the bad feelings and dedicate ourselves to being the best person possible. Don't let negative feelings or negative people eat you up.

There are a lot of valuable resources out there and many of them are free or low cost. There are many good people out there that care and are real "miracle" workers.

Remember always smile! Yes, I'm talking to you, the reader, and to the contributing authors of this book.

Smile...You are Beautiful!

Kathy Cournan Sarro

ABOUT KATHY COURNAN SARRO

Kathleen Cournan Sarro is a very humble mother of three beautiful boys. She has cared for children with special needs for almost 29 years. Known as an 'eternal optimist', she is passionate about helping people find hope when things feel hopeless. She helps others rise above some of their toughest challenges so they can reach their God-given potential. Being compassionate, loving, and non-judgmental are some of Kathleen's many gifts.

For the last twenty years, Kathleen has worked as a Certified Recreation Therapist Specialist (CTRS). In 2007, she became a Nurse Practitioner and uses her profession to help people be the best possible version of themselves. She has worked directly with people suffering from addiction for over ten years. She specialized in MAT (Medication Assisted Treatment), which includes Methadone, Suboxone, Subutex, Sublocade, and Vivitrol. She is also an advocate of people using other strategies such as their faith in God, Buddha, Alcoholics Anonymous, Narcotics Anonymous, and going cold turkey! Her motto is "do whatever works for you, as you are unique". She knows deep down that, in the end, love wins! Smile, you are beautiful!

Made in the USA
Las Vegas, NV
31 March 2023